T0294595

Gender Facial Affirmation Surgery

Editor

ANTHONY BARED

FACIAL PLASTIC SURGERY CLINICS OF NORTH AMERICA

www.facialplastic.theclinics.com

Consulting Editor
ANTHONY P. SCLAFANI

August 2023 • Volume 31 • Number 3

ELSEVIER

1600 John F. Kennedy Boulevard ● Suite 1800 ● Philadelphia, Pennsylvania, 19103-2899

http://www.theclinics.com

FACIAL PLASTIC SURGERY CLINICS OF NORTH AMERICA Volume 31, Number 3
August 2023 ISSN 1064-7406, ISBN-13: 978-0-443-18260-0

Editor: Stacy Eastman
Developmental Editor: Ann Gielou M. Posedio

Facial Plastic Surgery Clinics of North America (ISSN 1064-7406) is published quarterly by Elsevier Inc., 360 Park Avenue South, New York, NY 10010-1710. Months of issue are February, May, August, and November. Business and Editorial Offices: 1600 John F. Kennedy Blvd., Suite 1800, Philadelphia, PA 19103-2899. Periodicals postage paid at New York, NY, and additional mailing offices. Subscription prices are $428.00 per year (US individuals), $728.00 per year (US institutions), $477.00 per year (Canadian individuals), $904.00 per year (Canadian institutions), $568.00 per year (foreign individuals), $904.00 per year (foreign institutions), $100.00 per year (US students), $100.00 per year (Canadian students), and $255.00 per year (foreign students). Foreign air speed delivery is included in all *Clinics* subscription prices. All prices are subject to change without notice. POSTMASTER: Send address changes to *Facial Plastic Surgery Clinics*, Elsevier Health Sciences Division, Subscription Customer Service, 3251 Riverport Lane, Maryland Heights, MO 63043. **Customer service: 1-800-654-2452 (US and Canada); 1-314-447-8871 (outside US and Canada); Fax: 314-447-8029; E-mail: journalscustomerservice-usa@elsevier.com (for print support); journalsonlinesupport-usa@elsevier.com (for online support).**

Reprints. For copies of 100 or more of articles in this publication, please contact the Commercial Reprints Department, Elsevier Inc., 360 Park Avenue South, New York, NY 10010-1710. Tel.: 212-633-3874; Fax: 212-633-3820; E-mail: reprints@elsevier.com.

Facial Plastic Surgery Clinics of North America is covered in *MEDLINE/PubMed* (*Index Medicus*).

Contributors

CONSULTING EDITOR

ANTHONY P. SCLAFANI, MD, MBA, FACS
Director of Facial Plastic Surgery, Professor of
Otolaryngology- Head & Neck Surgery, Weill
Cornell Medical College, New York, New York

EDITOR

ANTHONY BARED, MD, FACS
Private Practice, Facial Plastic Surgery and
Hair Restoration, Miami, Florida

AUTHORS

BRANDON ALBA, MD
Resident, Division of Plastic and
Reconstructive Surgery, Rush University,
Affirm: The Rush Center for Gender, Sexuality
and Reproductive Health

ANTHONY BARED, MD, FACS
Private Practice, Facial Plastic Surgery and
Hair Restoration, Miami, Florida

JASON D. BLOOM, MD, FACS
Department of Otorhinolaryngology, University
of Pennsylvania, Philadelphia, Pennsylvania;
Bloom Facial Plastic Surgery, Bryn Mawr,
Pennsylvania

CARLY CLARK, MD
University of Kentucky Otolaryngology–Head
and Neck Surgery, Division of Facial Plastic
and Reconstructive Surgery, Lexington,
Kentucky

LANE DONALDSON, MD
Department of Otolaryngology, Henry Ford
Health, Detroit, Michigan

AMIR DORAFSHAR, MBChB, FAAP
Chair, Division of Plastic and Reconstructive
Surgery, Rush University, Affirm: The Rush
Center for Gender, Sexuality and Reproductive
Health

JEFFREY S. EPSTEIN, MD
Private Practice, Facial Plastic Surgery and
Hair Restoration, Miami, Florida

RUSSELL E. ETTINGER, MD
Assistant Professor, Division of Plastic
Surgery, Department of Surgery, University of
Washington, Division of Craniofacial and
Plastic Surgery, Department of Surgery,
Seattle Children's Hospital

ANNA J. FLAHERTY, MD
Facial Plastic and Reconstructive Surgery,
Division of Otolaryngology–Head and Neck
Surgery, Virginia Mason Medical Center,
Seattle, Washington

LAURA GARCIA-RODRIGUEZ, MD
Department of Otolaryngology, Henry Ford
Health, Detroit, Michigan

NIKITA GUPTA, MD
Assistant Professor, University of Kentucky
Otolaryngology–Head and Neck Surgery,
Division of Facial Plastic and Reconstructive
Surgery, Lexington, Kentucky

JACOB E. KUPERSTOCK, MD
Department of Facial Plastic and
Reconstructive Surgery, Otolaryngology
Associates, PC, Fairfax, Virginia

BENJAMIN B. MASSENBURG, MD
Resident in Plastic Surgery, Division of Plastic Surgery, Department of Surgery, University of Washington, Division of Craniofacial and Plastic Surgery, Department of Surgery, Seattle Children's Hospital

SHANE D. MORRISON, MD, MS
Assistant Professor, Division of Plastic Surgery, Department of Surgery, University of Washington, Division of Craniofacial and Plastic Surgery, Department of Surgery, Seattle Children's Hospital

MICHAEL J. NUARA, MD
Facial Plastic and Reconstructive Surgery, Division of Otolaryngology–Head and Neck Surgery, Virginia Mason Medical Center, Seattle, Washington

FEJIRO OKIFO, MD
Department of Otolaryngology, Henry Ford Health, Detroit, Michigan

MICHAL JAKUB PLOCIENNICZAK, MD, MSc
Department of Otolaryngology–Head and Neck Surgery, Division of Facial Plastic and Reconstructive Surgery, Boston University School of Medicine, Boston, Massachusetts; The Spiegel Center, Newton, Massachusetts

REGINA E. RODMAN, MD
Face Forward Houston, Houston, Texas

NAHIR J. ROMERO, MD
Somenek + Pittman MD Advanced Plastic Surgery, Washington, DC

LOREN SCHECHTER, MD, FACS
Division of Plastic and Reconstructive Surgery, Rush University, Director of Affirm: The Rush Center for Gender, Sexuality and Reproductive Health

MICHAEL SOMENEK, MD
Facial Plastic Surgeon, Facial Plastic Surgery, Somenek + Pittman MD Advanced Plastic Surgery, Washington, DC

JEFFREY HOWARD SPIEGEL, MD, FACS
Department of Otolaryngology–Head and Neck Surgery, Division of Facial Plastic and Reconstructive Surgery, Boston University School of Medicine, Boston, Massachusetts; The Spiegel Center, Newton, Massachusetts

ARI M. STONE, MD
Department of Otolaryngology–Head and Neck Surgery, Southern Illinois University, Springfield, Illinois

JEFFREY C. TEIXEIRA, MD, MBA
Uniformed Services University of the Health Science, Bethesda, Maryland

KATHERINE NICOLE VANDENBERG, MD
Department of Otolaryngology–Head and Neck Surgery, Division of Facial Plastic and Reconstructive Surgery, Boston University School of Medicine, Boston, Massachusetts; The Spiegel Center, Newton, Massachusetts

MAGGIE WANHE WANG, BA
Face Forward Houston, Houston, Texas

BRIELLE WEINSTEIN, MD
Clinical Instructor, Division of Plastic and Reconstructive Surgery, Rush University, Affirm: The Rush Center for Gender, Sexuality and Reproductive Health

ANNI WONG, MD
Department of Otorhinolaryngology, University of Pennsylvania, Philadelphia, Pennsylvania

GRACE T. WU, MD
Department of Otorhinolaryngology, University of Pennsylvania, Philadelphia, Pennsylvania

Contents

There are anthropometric differences between the bony and integumentary facial features of male and female individuals. When compared to males, female faces in general are more heart-shaped, with a shorter and smoother forehead, a smaller more defined nose, and a tapered chin.

Preparing for facial feminization surgery (FFS) or gender-affirming facial surgery is a daunting task. Patients do extensive research online to see what FFS means. Oftentimes it is the patients who are educating their physicians when discussing medical clearance or the esteemed "therapy letter." The therapy letter is a letter that details the support for surgery in a stable patient and reaffirms the need to have FFS in a person diagnosed with gender dysphoria. This typically follows the World Professional Association for Transgender Health standards-of-care guidelines. Besides having the therapy letter, patients must be counseled on concurrent mental health illnesses.

 Video content accompanies this article at http://www.facialplastic.theclinics.com.

Chondrolaryngoplasty is a surgical procedure that reduces the prominence of the thyroid notch. Although frequently performed on transgender (man to woman) women, anyone wishing to reduce the prominence of their thyroid notch for aesthetic purposes may consider undergoing a chondrolaryngoplasty. Direct visualization of the vocal cords with flexible laryngoscopy and intraoperative needle localization of the anterior commissure directs the extent of resection, helps increase safety, and avoids devastating postoperative voice complications. This procedure can be safely performed in combination with other facial feminization surgeries.

The upper third of the face has an important effect on gendering patients. Forehead contouring modifying a masculine face to a more feminine form is most likely to affect the gender assessment of an individual's face. Contouring involves techniques such as forehead reduction or augmentation, orbital contouring, and hairline adjustment. Traditionally, surgeons have utilized an open technique, though newer innovations such as endoscopic procedures and custom implants provide an alternative for patients with mild defects. Forehead contouring procedures are well tolerated with minimal side effects reported despite the proximity to the frontal sinus and cranial vault.

FACIAL PLASTIC SURGERY CLINICS OF NORTH AMERICA

SERIES OF RELATED INTEREST

Clinics in Plastic Surgery
https://www.plasticsurgery.theclinics.com
Otolaryngologic Clinics
https://www.oto.theclinics.com
Dermatologic Clinics
https://www.derm.theclinics.com
Advances in Cosmetic Surgery
https://www.advancesincosmeticsurgery.com/

THE CLINICS ARE AVAILABLE ONLINE!
Access your subscription at:
www.theclinics.com

Foreword
Gender Facial Affirmation Surgery

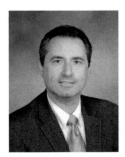

Anthony P. Sclafani, MD, MBA, FACS
Consulting Editor

> *You could leave life right now. Let that determine what you do and say and think.*
> —*Marcus Aurelius Antoninus,* **Meditations**

Marcus Aurelius (121-180 CE) wrote these words nearly 2 millennia ago, in his very personal explorations, "**Meditations**." At the pinnacle of power in control of one of the largest empires of antiquity, Marcus wrote these words to help himself navigate military challenges, palace intrigue, and the choices available to the most powerful person on earth at the time.

In this issue of *Facial Plastic Surgery Clinics of North America*, Anthony Bared, MD has assembled a stellar group of authors with extensive experience in gender-affirming care. Here you will find a compendium of facial plastic surgery techniques of both facial masculinization and feminization. Experienced authors comprehensively describe individualized treatments. We thank the authors for their clear descriptions of the indications and the nuances of these techniques. Gender-affirming care may elicit strong feelings on many sides, and you, dear reader, may choose not to perform this. But it is worthwhile also to contemplate these words of Marcus:

> *Every living organism is fulfilled when it follows the right path for its own nature.*
> —*Marcus Aurelius Antoninus,* **Meditations**

Anthony P. Sclafani, MD, MBA, FACS
Department of Otolaryngology
Weill Cornell Medicine
Weill Greenberg Center
1305 York Avenue, Suite Y-5
New York, NY 10021, USA

E-mail address:
ans9243@med.cornell.edu

Facial Plast Surg Clin N Am 31 (2023) ix
https://doi.org/10.1016/j.fsc.2023.05.001
1064-7406/23/© 2023 Published by Elsevier Inc.

Preface
Techniques and Perspectives in Facial Gender Affirmation Surgery

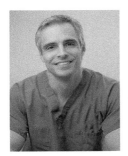

Anthony Bared, MD, FACS
Editor

Gender dysphoria has been a topic of increasing awareness in recent years. Gender dysphoria affects individuals whose gender assigned at birth does not align with their gender identity. Persistent identification with the opposite gender can result in significant stress and impairment leading to an increased rate of depression, anxiety, and suicide in individuals with gender dysphoria versus the general population. Facial gender modification is often sought by individuals with gender dysphoria to help align their external appearance with the gender they identify with internally, helping to improve quality of life.

In this issue, we have brought together a group of experts in the field of facial gender affirmation surgery to provide a comprehensive review of different surgical and nonsurgical modalities to help in our care of the gender-dysmorphic patient seeking facial transitioning procedures. Our experts discuss facial gender affirmation surgery as it pertains to facial feminization and facial masculinization procedures. We present a spectrum of procedures to help those physicians providing facial gender affirmation surgical and nonsurgical procedures hone their own techniques and provide them with tools to optimize their patient's care.

Anthony Bared, MD, FACS
Facial Plastic Surgery and Hair Restoration
6280 Sunset Drive
Suite 506
Miami, FL 33143, USA

E-mail address:
abared@dranthonybared.com

Facial Plast Surg Clin N Am 31 (2023) xi
https://doi.org/10.1016/j.fsc.2023.04.007
1064-7406/23/© 2023 Published by Elsevier Inc.

Facial Analysis for Gender Affirmation/Gender-Related Facial Analysis

Michael Somenek, MD[a],*, Nahir J. Romero, MD[b]

KEYWORDS

• Gender facial analysis • Gender-affirming surgery • Esthetic anthropometry

KEY POINTS

• Historically, there are known anthropometric variances between the skeleton as well as the soft tissues of male and female individuals.
• It is important to recognize the characteristic differences between male and female faces to achieve desirable results during gender affirmation interventions.
• Facial canons are more artistic perceptions and not realistic when analyzing facial morphological differences.
• A more standardized method should be established to approach facial analysis on patients with gender dysphoria.

INTRODUCTION

As gender dysphoria becomes more recognized and medical insurances start covering surgical gender affirmation procedures, the term and surgical options for treatment have become more known and recognized among the surgical community. For this reason, more publications and reports are being written describing surgical techniques, outcomes, safety, and patient satisfaction.

It is estimated that there are at least 1.5 million transgender individuals in the United States and most agree this estimate is low. There has been an overall increased demand for facial feminization procedures to treat gender dysphoria. In the past 5 to 7 years, some institutions have reported a 13-fold increase in requests for facial feminization procedures.[1]

Some have proposed that this increase in demand can be related to the elements of facial social recognition and how this affects people's daily lives. Studies have shown that the mental health and quality of life of these individuals can

be greatly diminished.[2] However, these greatly improve once they have undergone their facial feminization surgery (FFS) reporting high levels of satisfaction after FFS.[3]

Despite the increasingly growing number of gender-affirming surgical interventions, little can be found in descriptions between feminine and masculine morphologic differences. Additionally, there is also a lack of strategic or standardized ways on how to successfully address these differences.

The facial morphologic features that identify a face as masculine or feminine are diverse and complex. In this article, we attempt to provide a logical and systematic method of facial analysis so providers can have a well-informed discussion with their patients preoperatively.

History

When it comes to cosmetic surgery, true proportions are assessed using anthropometric techniques, which work as a guide to correct facial deformities or disproportions.

[a] Facial Plastic Surgery, Somenek+PittmanMD Advanced Plastic Surgery, 2440 M Street Northwest Suite 507, Washington, DC 20037, USA; [b] Somenek +Pittman MD, 2440 M Street Northwest Suite 507, Washington, DC 20037, USA
* Corresponding author.
E-mail address: msomenek@gmail.com

Facial Plast Surg Clin N Am 31 (2023) 341–348
https://doi.org/10.1016/j.fsc.2023.03.002
1064-7406/23/© 2023 Elsevier Inc. All rights reserved.

Measurements of the human face have been performed since ancient Greek times. Many aspects of measurements established during that time can still be found in contemporary clinical anthropometry.

During these early times, human forms and canons were represented based on the preference of the artist, rather than how they objectively and realistically were. Greek artists wanted to identify ideal facial proportions and began to analyze beauty in a formal way. The classical canons of facial balance that they developed consequently influenced anatomic scholars of the Renaissance period.[4]

Aristotle described the science of reading one's character from one's bodily features.[5] Interestingly, he compared male and female features to those of various animals. He found male individuals to look like brave lions because of the larger mouth, squarer face, equally balanced jaws, bright, deep-set eyes, large eyebrows, and square forehead. In his opinion, based on their features, women were more like shy panthers. To Aristotle, beauty meant symmetry, harmony, and geometry.[6]

Leonardo da Vinci extensively reported on body and facial proportions and how they ideally should be shaped. He applied these canons in his art during the Renaissance period. Even though he dictated these strict canons, he could not deny the natural variations in nature from one person to another after taking and comparing measurements from live bodies.

Albrecht Durer, a German painter, also felt a system of canons could be implemented to define the ideal proportions for human bodies and faces, making them result in the most beautiful figures.[1,7] After some trialing with sizes and proportions, he (like da Vinci), established that the face was divided into three equal lengths: the forehead, the nose, and the mouth/chin.[4,8] He also found that the width between the eyes equaled the size of one eye.[6] Durer felt deviations from his canons were unesthetic, however, most of the heads he painted are unattractive to the general public's eyes.[7]

Anthropometrist Leslie Farkas challenged these classic canons by measuring the facial proportions of 200 women, including 50 models.[9] His results concluded, as we suspected, some of the ancient canons are nothing more than artistic idealizations. Nevertheless, these esthetic canons have withstood the test of time, even with the social and cultural influences every generation holds about the concept of beauty. Currently, the parameters established in the facial plastic surgery literature are based predominately on the works of

Powell and Humphreys,[10] who in 1984 solidified this topic into their text, Proportions of the Aesthetic Face.[6]

Facial Analysis

Facial analysis is crucial for surgical planning and a fundamental element when evaluating a patient for any facial plastic cosmetic or reconstructive surgical intervention. A systematic assessment allows the surgeon to identify harmony, proportions, and balance to determine if these are esthetically pleasing based on general anthropometric guides and measurements.

Facial analysis is dependent on soft tissue as well as skeletal anatomic landmarks. When we talk about soft tissue references, some of the most important points of reference include the trichion, radix, subnasale, the superior and inferior vermilion border, stomion, and the menton. Skeletal reference points are defined by cephalometric analysis, some of which include the sella, orbitale, the anterior nasal spine, subspinale, prosthion, pogonion, gnathion, and the gonion[6] (Table 1).

Utilizing these standard points of origin, reference angles have been created to better understand and analyze interfacial relationships. Although they serve as a general orientation, it is important to remember that gender and ethnic variations exist. Men typically have sharper angles and more prominent features when compared to women. It is these variations that help us recognize gender, as well as the degree of femininity and masculinity in a subconscious way.[5]

There are also different methods to systematically analyze a facial appearance. The first method divides the face into equal thirds as described by da Vinci. Measurements are taken in the midline, from the trichion to the glabella (forehead and brow), from the glabella to the subnasale (orbits, cheeks, and nose), and from the subnasale to the menton (lips, mandible, and chin) (Fig. 1).

A different technique is utilized at times, discounting the upper third of the face due to the common inconsistencies in hairline position. Measurements are made from the nasion (instead of the glabella) to the subnasale and from the subnasale to the menton.[6] Generally speaking, the female skull is smaller and rounder than the male skull. The female skull also has a greater projection of the zygomatic prominences that softly taper into a slimmer chin. This makes the female face possess a more heart-shaped appearance when compared to a more square male face.[11,12]

Another way of dividing the face for analysis is doing vertical fifths. The width of each individual eye is one-fifth of the facial width and should be

Table 1
Skeletal cephalometric reference points

Skeletal Cephalometric Reference Points	
Sella	Midpoint of the hypophysial fossa
Orbitale	Most inferior point on the infraorbital rim
Porion	Most superior point on external auditory meatus
Condylion	Most superior point on the head of the mandibular condyle
Articulate	Point of intersection of the posterior margin of the ascending mandibular ramus and the outer margin of the cranial base
Anterior nasal spine	Projection of the maxilla at the base of the nose
Posterior nasal spine	Medial end of the posterior palatine bone process projection
Subspinale	Deepest point in the concavity of the premaxilla
Prosthion	Lowest, most anterior point on the alveolar portion of the premaxilla
Infradentale	Highest, most anterior point on the alveolar portion of the mandible
Supramentale	Most posterior point in the outer contour of the mandibular alveolar process
Pogonion	Most anterior point on the bony chin in the midline
Gnathion	Point between the most anterior (pogonion) and inferior (menton) points on the chin
Menton	Lowest point on the mandible
Gonion	Midpoint at the angle of the mandible

equal to the intercanthal distance. The remaining two-fifths are measured from the lateral canthus of the eye to the helix of each ear.

When analyzing a face for facial feminization or masculinization, it is helpful to perform the evaluation in a methodical way to better understand the balance and proportions for the given gender affirmation surgery. In an effort to create some standardization to the facial analysis process, we will break down the analysis of the face into thirds: upper, middle, and lower.

Upper Third

When evaluating the upper third of the face, some of the more important features include the shape of the hairline, the length and convexity of the forehead, bossing of the supraorbital area, glabella, and the position of the brow.

When it comes to hairlines, a feminine hairline is smoothly contoured and fuller. Masculine hairlines tend to have a widow's peak, be M shaped, and at times can be receding due to a higher incidence of androgenetic alopecia.[12,13] The distance from the nasion to the hairline is usually shorter in females by about 1 cm (**Fig. 2**).

The boundaries of the forehead are from the hairline to the glabella. The contour of the forehead anatomy is esthetically pleasing when there is a gentle convexity on the profile. A line tangent to the glabella through the nasion and intersecting with a line tangent to the nasal dorsum creates the nasofrontal angle which ranges from 115° to 135°. It is usually more acute in males and more obtuse in females. The supraorbital ridge is more prominent in men and tends to blend medially into the glabella which gives it a more projected appearance. This is viewed as a more masculine trait.

When comparing female and male characteristics, male individuals have a flatter appearance to their forehead, with more pronounced supraorbital ridges, and a less steep slant from the ridge to the vertex. They can possess some bossing and a prominent anterior convexity. The frontal sinus development in male individuals contributes to this and can also produce a discontinuous curvature. The female forehead is vertically higher, with a softer, gentler arch (**Fig. 3**).

The brow begins in a slight clublike shape medially and continues in a gradual taper toward its lateral end. In female, it starts medially below the supraorbital rim or at the rim then arches up as it moves laterally until it peaks at the lateral third. The lateral position in female individuals is well above the supraorbital rim. The male brow is straighter, thicker, and usually lays right at the level or very close to the supraorbital rim.

The medial edge of the eyebrow rests on a perpendicular line that extends from the lateral-most portion of the nasal ala and about 10 mm above the medial canthus. In female individuals, the highest point of the eyebrow arch is at a line drawn through the lateral limbus. However, this idyllic position can vary with fashion trends. The actual zenith's highest point may lie in any place from the lateral canthus to the lateral limbus.

The limits of the orbits are in the lower third of the upper face reaching into the upper third of

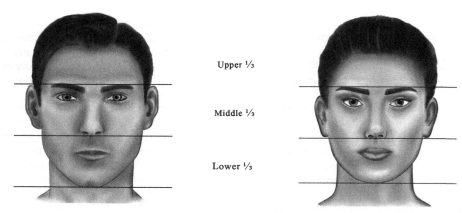

Fig. 1. The face is divided into horizontal thirds which provides the foundation for proper understanding and analysis of proportions.

the midface. As previously mentioned with the rule of fifths, the width of one eye from medial to lateral canthus should equal one-fifth of the facial width and the intercanthal distance should equal this measurement as well. Average intercanthal distances are 25.5 to 37.5 mm and 26.5 to 38.7 mm for women and men, respectively.[6] In comparative proportions, when evaluating the overall facial mass, the female orbits are larger and appear in a slightly higher position on the skull.[8]

Middle Third

When analyzing the middle third of the face, the areas that must be considered are the orbital and periorbital tissue, the zygomatic arches, and the nose.

The female orbits as previously mentioned are usually larger, rounder, and higher placed, but their upper and lateral portions appear less prominent than in males. When it comes to eyelids, the female eyelid crease is usually positioned higher with a maximum distance of 12 mm from the lid margin (compared to 8 mm in males). Male upper

eyelids appear to have more volume with less pretarsal show that can create a slightly heavier appearance to the eyelid.[4] The canthal lean or angle is slightly more positive in female individuals.[4,7] There are very minimal differences when it comes to lower eyelids between male and female individuals. Women appear to have augmented periorbital soft tissue luminosity, which is likely the result of reduced dermal thickness. This provides a more youthful look with a less recessed appearance and should be taken into account and addressed as well.[11,14]

The boundaries of the nose are within the middle third of the face and all of its subdivisions need to be taken into account including the dorsum, tip, and alar base.

When it comes to the nose, male nasal bones tend to be larger and meet at a sharper angle at the midline.[8] The nasal aperture is narrower and higher with sharp margins instead of rounded. These will result in the male nose having a more noticeable dorsal spine and squarer at the base. They also have a broader alar width. Female noses on the other hand are shorter and smaller,

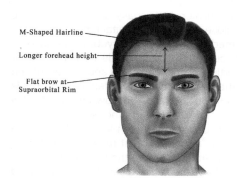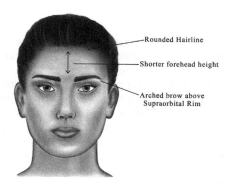

Fig. 2. Key differences between the upper third of the face are shown in males (*Left*) and females (*right*).

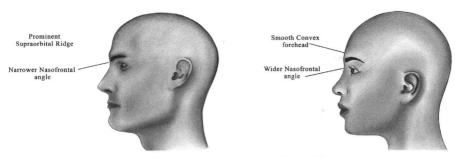

Fig. 3. The prominent supraorbital ridge is a key feature in a male face while the wider nasofrontal angle is more common in females.

with narrower alar bases and bridges. The nasolabial angle defines the angular inclination of the columella as it encounters the upper lip. The angle is formed between the connection of a line tangent to the labrale superius and subnasale, and a line tangent to the subnasale and the most anterior point of the columella. This angle should measure 95° to 110° in women and 90° to 95° in men, being more obtuse in female individuals.[12] When it comes to the nose, it is considered more attractive in female to have a more defined tip and a straight dorsum.[11] There is a significant difference in the labial insertion of the alar base between male and female individuals. This results in a larger nasal width-to-lip ratio in male individuals.

As stated previously, ethnic and facial variations can impact facial proportions, as this is especially true when addressing the nose. Therefore, it is imperative to keep this in mind when deciding how the nasal appearance and position are addressed during a gender-affirming surgery.

When talking about the zygomatic regions (cheekbones), they are usually stronger and heavier in men. In contrast, the malar bones are more prominent in women, but refined and lighter.[4] This increased fullness in the maxillary area when compared to the mandibular angle in females is what gives their faces that characteristic heart shape appearance (**Fig. 4**).

The interzygomatic width is the distance measured by a line between the most prominent points of the zygomatic arch on both sides of the face. Anthropometric studies have revealed this distance is meaningfully higher in male when compared to female individuals.[15] That proportion in female individuals creates a facial taper that gives the face a characteristic heart shape or tapered triangular appearance from the upper third to the lower third of the face. The taper from this line is thought to be associated with a more feminine and attractive appearance. The role of mandibular sculpting is reducing this bigonial width relative to the interzygomatic distance to help achieve a more feminine look (**Fig. 5**).

Lower Third

When discussing the lower third of the face, the more prominent features include the vermilion, gonial angle, mandible, and the chin. In women, the upper lip length is shorter with fuller volume and a well-formed cupid's bow.[12] The vermilion and cutaneous portions of the lower lip are almost equal in thickness. A more masculine-appearing lip has a thinner vermilion border, which is the red portion of the lip, as well as a longer upper

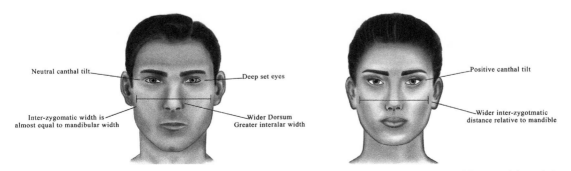

Fig. 4. The middle third of the face is different between men and women in the orbital, nasal base width and tip, as well as the zygomatic prominences.

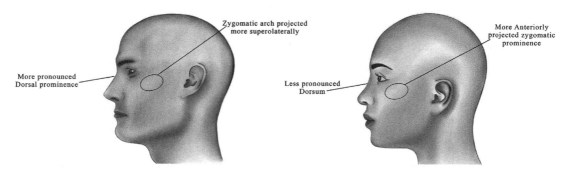

Fig. 5. The position and highlight of the zygomatic arch is projected more superolaterally in a male and more anteriorly in the female.

cutaneous lip portion, which is formed by the skin portion that goes from the nasal sill and columella down to the vermilion border. To obtain facial balance, the vertical upper lip length from the stomion to the subnasale should be one-third of the lower facial third, and the lower lip and chin from the menton to the stomion will constitute the other two-thirds. Having a shorter cutaneous portion of the lip will provide more vermilion show and change the lip width and profile appearance to a higher, more pouty look. This can be evaluated by drawing a line from the subnasale to the pogonion. The most anterior aspect of the upper lip should lie 3.5 mm anterior to the line and the lower lip 2.2 mm.[4] This is not only associated with femininity but also with youth. It can also allow for a small amount of maxillary teeth show, which can be esthetically pleasing. The height of the white upper lip has been found to be bigger in male than female individuals. A longer cutaneous portion of the lip can give the appearance of a longer, flatter lip that can sometimes hide or decrease vermilion show by curling inward. This has been associated with a more masculine appearance.

Surgical methods like lip lift, corner lift, and dermal grafts can be implemented to help achieve a shorter cutaneous lip height and increase the vermilion show, providing a more feminine look. They can also be combined with filler to provide additional volume and pout once the vermilion show of the lip has been increased.

The mandible in men is dimensionally thicker and larger, with greater body height and more prominent gonial angles, giving it a squarer appearance.[16] Owing to the mandibular attachments, it is usually heavier, taller, and wider.[17] The angle of the mandible should be well-defined and sharp. In contrast, women have a more obtuse gonial angle. This gives the female jaw a softer, more curved appearance, with a narrower mandibular width. The transition from the body to the ramus tends to be smoother[8] (**Fig. 6**).

When evaluating the chin, males typically have a longer, more projected chin compared to females by as much as 20%. The shape is squarer in males and more trapezoidal in females.[17] Women usually have a single medial mental eminence, making the chin more rounded or pointier, with an overall more tapered appearance.[7,11] When the chin is in line with the lower lip vermilion or slightly anterior,

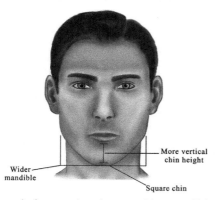
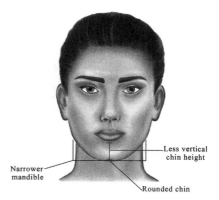

Fig. 6. The male face tends to have a wider mandible and more pronounced and square chin. The female face is usually more tapered with a narrower mandible and rounded chin.

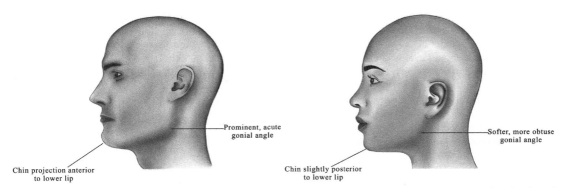

Prominent, acute
gonial angle

Softer, more obtuse
gonial angle

Chin projection anterior
to lower lip

Chin slightly posterior
to lower lip

Fig. 7. Males have a more projected chin anterior to the lower lip with a more acute gonial angle. The female gonial angle is more obtuse with less chin projection.

this is considered a more masculinizing characteristic (**Fig. 7**).

Occlusion and dentition are very important factors to take into consideration as well as the use of orthodontia. This can mask and/or modify a non-harmonious relationship between the nose, the lip, and the chin and should always be discussed with the patient.

Soft Tissue Considerations

When we consider skin and integument tissues, in general, male skin is thicker when compared to females. Also, male skin has less subcutaneous fat and tissue present, likely due to hair follicles and their supporting structures along the dermis under the influence of testosterone. In contrast, female structures under the stimuli of estrogen possess a greater amount of subcutaneous fat, which will result in a more feminine contour.[18]

In addition, an important factor to consider is the aging process of your particular patient. Males and females age differently with particularly noticeable changes along the mandible and the brow area. If these are considered preemptively, attention can be taken to address these particular areas during the same surgical intervention and prevent these aging changes to masculinize the face.

Other important considerations that can help enhance and complete your planning and maximize your surgical results are the patient's quality and texture of their skin, hairstyle, facial hair, brow, lashes, facial fat, and facial volume. Based on the results of your evaluation, supplementary options can be offered to optimize the surgical results. Facial hair patterns should be observed and different hair removal strategies should be discussed like laser or electrolysis. Taking all of these into account can have a major effect and ultimately maximize the overall esthetic for a particular patient.

SUMMARY

There are recognizable anthropometric differences between feminine and masculine facial features. A standardized method of evaluating these critical differences is necessary when counseling patients before facial gender affirmation surgery. They will help set goals preoperatively between patient and surgeon as well as aid the surgeon with surgical planning. They can also help set post-operative expectations. FFS is a crucial step for patients looking to achieve congruency and harmony with their gender identity. Over the past few years, new studies have been completed on facial analysis to better understand and describe the differences between male and female faces.[19] These anthropometric differences between feminine and masculine faces are important for individuals to be properly identified in public as their preferred gender. We have described a systematic way to analyze these facial features by dividing and evaluating the face in thirds and highlighting each area's most important characteristics. This will provide the surgeon with a methodical way of examining all the different areas of the face and provide a more comprehensive and successful result.

DISCLOSURE

The authors have nothing to disclosures.

ACKNOWLEDGMENTS

Endless thanks to Kaitlin Tkac for her talented illustrations that beautifully complement the gender facial analysis descriptions.

REFERENCES

1. Tirrell AR, Abu El Hawa AA, Bekeny JC, et al. Facial Feminization Surgery: A Systematic Review of

Perioperative Surgical Planning and Outcomes. Plast Reconstr Surg Glob Open 2022;10(3):e4210.

2. Ainsworth TA, Spiegel JH. Quality of life of individuals with and without facial feminization surgery or gender reassignment surgery. Qual Life Res 2010;19(7):1019–24.

3. Pavlidis L, Spyropoulou GA, Dionyssiou D, et al. Full Facial Feminization Surgery: Patient Satisfaction Assessment Based on 180 Procedures Involving 33 Consecutive Patients. Plast Reconstr Surg 2016;138(4):765e–6e.

4. Bailey BJ, Johnson JT, Rosen CA. Bailey's head and neck surgery - otolaryngology preoperative evaluation and facial analysis in facial plastic surgery. Philadelphia, PA: Wolters Kluwer, Lippincott Williams et Wilkins; 2014.

5. Spiegel JH. Challenges in care of the transgender patient seeking facial feminization surgery. Facial Plast Surg Clin North Am 2008;16(2):233, viii.

6. Flint PW, Zimbler MS. Aesthetic facial analysis/facial plastic and reconstructive surgery. Cummings Otolaryngology–Head & Neck Surgery. Philadelphia: Elsevier/Saunders; 2015. p. 236–47.

7. Vegter F, Hage JJ. Clinical anthropometry and canons of the face in historical perspective. Plast Reconstr Surg 2000;106(5):1090–6.

8. Becking AG, Tuinzing DB, Hage JJ, et al. Transgender feminization of the facial skeleton. Clin Plast Surg 2007;34(3):557–64.

9. Rodman R. Developments in facial feminization surgery. Curr Opin Otolaryngol Head Neck Surg 2022;30(4):249–53.

10. Chaya BF, Berman ZP, Boczar D, et al. Current Trends in Facial Feminization Surgery: An Assessment of Safety and Style. J Craniofac Surg 2021;32(7):2366–9.

11. Hage JJ, Becking AG, de Graaf FH, et al. Gender-confirming facial surgery: considerations on the masculinity and femininity of faces. Plast Reconstr Surg 1997;99(7):1799–807.

12. Sedgh. The Aesthetics of the Upper Face and Brow: Male and Female Differences. Facial Plast Surg 2018;34(2):114–8.

13. Salman KE, Altunay IK, Kucukunal NA, et al. Frequency, severity and related factors of androgenetic alopecia in dermatology outpatient clinic: hospital-based cross-sectional study in Turkey. An Bras Dermatol 2017;92(1):35–40.

14. Ousterhout DK. Feminization of the forehead: contour changing to improve female aesthetics. Plast Reconstr Surg 1987;79(5):701–13.

15. Moreno Uribe LM, Ray A, Blanchette DR, et al. Phenotype-genotype correlations of facial width and height proportions in patients with Class II malocclusion. Orthod Craniofac Res 2015;18 Suppl 1(0 1):100–8.

16. Altman K. Facial feminization surgery: current state of the art. Int J Oral Maxillofac Surg 2012;41(8):885–94.

17. Powell N, Humphreys B. Proportions of the aesthetic face. New York: Thieme-Stratton; 1984.

18. Raffaini, Magri AS, Agostini T. Full Facial Feminization Surgery: Patient Satisfaction Assessment Based on 180 Procedures Involving 33 Consecutive Patients. Plast Reconstr Surg 2016;137(2):438–48.

19. Bannister JJ, Juszczak H, Aponte JD, et al. Sex Differences in Adult Facial Three-Dimensional Morphology: Application to Gender-Affirming Facial Surgery. Facial Plast Surg Aesthet Med 2022;24(S2):S24–30.

Preparing for Facial Feminization Surgery

Lane Donaldson, MD, Fejiro Okifo, MD, Laura Garcia-Rodriguez, MD*

KEYWORDS

- Facial feminization surgery (FFS) • Gender-affirming facial surgery (GAS)
- World Professional Association for Transgender Health (WPATH) • Hormones • Letter
- Gender dysphoria

KEY POINTS

- Facial feminization surgery (FFS) or gender-affirming facial surgery can help patients achieve congruence between their gender and their external appearance.
- Mental health providers will use World Professional Association for Transgender Health guidelines to help in writing a letter of support to those patients seeking surgery through an insurance pathway.
- Following recommendations of the guidelines, mental health professionals are able to write letters and specifically detail important patient history, including hormone length, societal transition, other mental health diagnosis, coping mechanisms, and any deterrents to a successful surgical outcome.
- Physicians and mental health providers should attempt to find patients who may have unrealistic expectations or those with other overlapping mental health diseases, such as body dysmorphic disorder.
- Patients who undergo FFS have to have clear expectations of postoperative outcomes.

INTRODUCTION

Facial surgery, including reconstructive and aesthetic, has certain implicit expectations. In cases of reconstructive surgery, the expectations are to create or restore function; however, this has shifted to create harmony and congruence in patients who have gender dysphoria. Gender dysphoria can be treated with multiple, interrelated modalities, including psychotherapy, hormone therapy, and surgical intervention. A combination of hormone therapy and surgical intervention can be necessary to reduce gender dysphoria in certain patients. Expectations for gender-affirming facial feminization surgery (FFS) can vary from patient to patient. Classically, the face has been divided into thirds or fifths, and other variations, to illustrate how different facial landmarks can create harmony.[1] There are ideal locations of eyebrows, nose width, and studies that note differences in the male versus female anatomy.[2] Some of this is used as a guide for affirming surgery, as not all rules fit everyone's face. For patients who are transgender, their features do not always align with their gender. The goal of FFS or gender-affirming facial surgery (GAS) is to create a more congruent aesthetic to the gender one is. Facial affirmation surgery does not necessarily mean the whole face will be different or mean a face transplant, but signs of excess testosterone can be reduced. This has to be discussed in depth.

FFS was pioneered by Douglas Ousterhout in the late 1980s as craniofacial surgery shifted focus to include addressing gender dysphoria.[3] This was borne out of the idea that there are underlying differences in the facial morphology between men and women. Ousterhout described surgeries to alter the forehead and jaws in order to more approximate a patient's intended gender.[3] The

Department of Otolaryngology, Henry Ford Health, Detroit, MI 48202, USA
* Corresponding author. ENT Clinic, 2nd Floor, West Wing, Henry Ford Hospital West Bloomfield, 6777 West Maple Road, West Bloomfield, MI 48322.
E-mail address: LGARCIA5@HFHS.ORG

Facial Plast Surg Clin N Am 31 (2023) 349–354
https://doi.org/10.1016/j.fsc.2023.03.004

umbrella of FFS includes but is not exclusive to feminization of the hairline and hair transplants, cranioplasty to reduce frontal bossing, rhinoplasty, lip augmentation surgery, genioplasty, mandibular contouring, and chondrolaryngoplasty in order to reduce the appearance of the Adam's apple. Because of variables between patients, the entire face may not need to be altered.

Transgender patients that are interested in GAS undergo a preoperative planning process that will sometimes include the collaboration of a multidisciplinary team, which is often in the academic setting. The team includes a patient's surgeon and may also include a primary care physician, an endocrinologist, and a mental health provider. Differences between surgeons in private practice and academic medicine will occur because those in private practice may cater to out-of-state patients where communication may be more limited. Because of this, therapy and health appraisal letters would be needed because the patient history may not be as easily accessible. The authors discuss the preoperative experience at their academic center in this article.

STAGED SURGERY

Completion of FFS can take different roads. A patient may choose to undergo surgery in stages or as a full-FFS procedure. The preoperative evaluation should include photographs taken during the clinic visit. Computed tomographic scans can also be useful in preoperative planning to plan the adjustment of the patient's masculine characteristics and also to identify variations in anatomic structures; however, this is not the standard of care. This is encouraged especially in patients who may have had facial trauma, tumors, or any congenital deformity.[4] However, the authors point out that it is not rare that patients will come in with CT scan images in hand.

Requests for a full FFS are much more common because there is only one recovery period. Full FFS refers to facial feminization surgery that "addresses the upper, middle, and lower facial thirds in a single anesthetic event."[5] Some of the surgeries that may be addressed include forehead cranioplasty, burring of the supraorbital ridge, blepharoplasty, rhinoplasty, upper lift lip, mandibular angle reduction, and tracheal shave. Single-stage FFS has not been shown to incur additional risk to the patient.[5] In addition, patients and physicians alike may be concerned about the infection risk in such lengthy cases or the fact that the surgeries are in different anatomic locations. Studies have shown that full FFS in different surgical planes (subperiosteal, subcutaneous, intraoral,

intranasal, and so forth) does not have an additive risk of infections.[6]

There is no consensus regarding the best practices for FFS. As previously discussed, staging surgeries is a patient-driven decision. At the authors' academic center, they limit surgeries to 8 hours of general anesthesia. A full-face surgery can be completed during that time. However, a small minority of patients decide to split these surgeries, or they may only desire a few of them owing to personal preference. Some surgeries are encouraged to be staged in cases of aggressive bony reduction followed by skin-tightening procedures. An example of a case where it is encouraged to split the case is in those patients who have a history of silicone injections and may have silicone granulomas (**Fig. 1**).[7] The silicone is removed to a variable amount, oftentimes leaving ptotic and volume lacking soft tissues. In the authors' institution, the silicone removal along with bony surgery is advocated followed by soft tissue work.

For some people, a staged approach is better after having an upfront discussion on the goals of surgery. Some preference may just be due to avoiding surgery that is longer than 8 hours, mostly owing to physician well-being and for patient safety. Some experts agree that staging surgery for some patients is advantageous if there is aggressive bony reduction that may leave "loose" skin, which can then be addressed with secondary tightening rejuvenation procedures. These can be then addressed at a mutually agreed upon time down the line with soft tissue modifications, such as fat grafting and manipulation of soft tissues via face lift or neck lift. In the authors' institution, it is customary for a minimum 6-month wait for the secondary skin-tightening procedures. As discussed before, it may be patient preference, as the

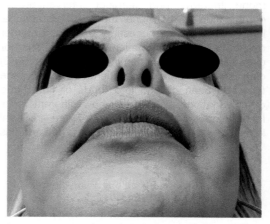

Fig. 1. Patient with noted silicone oil in the bilateral cheeks.

authors have had patients request surgery in blocks owing to fear of being under general anesthetic for longer than 3 hours. This has occurred with a few patients over the years. Extensive discussion must take place owing to the nature of being able to plan time away from family, work, or other responsibilities.

WORLD PROFESSIONAL ASSOCIATION FOR TRANSGENDER HEALTH

Preparing for FFS or GAS is a daunting task. Patients do extensive research online to see what FFS means. Oftentimes it is patients who are educating their physicians and other providers when discussing medical clearance or the esteemed "therapy letter." This is mostly an insurance requirement; however, each surgeon may need one depending on their personal evaluation of the patient. The therapy letter is a letter that details the support for surgery in a stable patient and reaffirms the need to have FFS in a person diagnosed with gender dysphoria. This typically follows the World Professional Association for Transgender Health (WPATH) standards-of-care guidelines.[8] Following recommendations of the guidelines, mental health professionals are able to write letters and specifically detail important patient history, including hormone length, societal transition, other mental health diagnosis, coping mechanisms, and any deterrents to a successful surgical outcome. Besides having the therapy letter, patients must be counseled on concurrent mental health illnesses, such as body dysmorphic disorder (BDD), to better understand the realistic postoperative outcome. Following extensive in-office or electronic discussion, scheduling the patient for surgery is done at a mutually convenient time, which allows for an appropriate recovery. Following surgery, some patients may benefit from additional therapy owing to the high incidence of depression.[9]

WORLD PROFESSIONAL ASSOCIATION FOR TRANSGENDER HEALTH PSYCHOLOGICAL LETTER

Before pursuing GAS, patients must undergo assessment by and provide referral letters from a mental health provider that is in accordance with the WPATH Standards of Care, 8th Version.[8] The WPATH has published several statements that serve as a guideline in the preoperative assessment of transgender and gender diverse (TGD) patients seeking GAS or other medical treatment. To qualify for GAS, the patient's gender incongruence must be marked and sustained in nature and can

be supported by factors, such as prior health care documentation, change in name and identity documents, and even open discussion about one's own gender. In addition, it is not necessary to have severe gender identity distress, as GAS can serve as a prophylactic means to prevent significant distress. The WPATH states that in regions where a specific diagnosis is necessary to access health care, a diagnosis of HA60 *Gender Incongruence of Adolescence or Adulthood* should be determined before gender-affirming interventions. Furthermore, preoperative evaluation should assess for other possible causes of apparent gender incongruence as well as identification of any additional mental health conditions that could adversely affect the GAS and postoperative care. Finally, an assessment for the patient's capacity to provide consent to GAS needs to be performed. Each patient's ability to understand the specific GAS, including risks and benefits, alternative treatments options, and potential short- and long-term consequences of the chosen GAS, needs to be assessed preoperatively.

HORMONES (LENGTH OF HORMONE TREATMENT)

In addition to the preoperative surgical assessment outlined by WPATH for GAS, hormone therapy is an important component in a patient's treatment and assessment before surgery.[8] Similar to GAS, eligible patients must meet all criteria as outlined previously in their pretreatment assessment. The goal for hormone therapy is to target serum levels of the sex steroids to match the levels associated with the individual's gender identity; however, there is no defined optimal range. Per the WPATH, initial treatment with hormone therapy should be followed by regular clinical evaluations for physical changes and potential adverse reactions to sex steroid hormones, including laboratory monitoring of sex steroid hormones every 3 months during the first year of hormone therapy or with dose changes until stable adult dosing is reached followed by clinical and laboratory testing once or twice a year once an adult maintenance dose is attained. Patients are generally required to be on hormone therapy for at least 6 months based on the new WPATH guidelines.[8] Current standards of care recommend cessation of hormone therapy for 1 to 4 weeks before surgery to minimize the risk of venous thromboembolism (VTE) associated with hormone therapy; however, these recommendations are not evidence-based and most commonly associated with genital surgery. Despite this, for patients who have already undergone gonadectomy, no studies have shown increased perioperative VTE while continuing hormone therapy, and the WPATH currently recommends continuing hormone therapy for these patients to avoid the adverse effects of discontinuing therapy. However, there is no clear large study analysis to understand the actual incidence in the transgender population.[10] To reiterate the individuality of each treatment plan, each surgeon, and patient, some elect to not stop hormones after having an educated decision, and also based on the fact that facial surgeon does not preclude patients from early mobilization.

SOCIETAL TRANSITION

For TGD patients pursuing GAS, societal transition often begins well before the decision to pursue surgery. The process can take months to years and often starts with questioning and exploring their identity as transgender, gender diverse, or gender nonbinary. Patients before and after GAS may present in public in their identified gender part-time or full-time. Public appearance can be altered in a multitude of ways, such as modifying wardrobes, use of make-up, and attire to modify appearance to the identified gender (eg, tight underwear or a gaff to obscure male genitalia and provide a female appearance or a binder to minimize the appearance of a female chest and appear more like that of a male chest). This again is fluid in nature because gender expression is also very fluid. The transition can be as public as announcing to partners, family, and friends or as private as keeping the transition to oneself. As part of this transition, patients may change their legal name or used pronouns. Patients may face significant discrimination from society and their peers, as well as from their local government, as not all communities recognize TGD patients in equal legal terms.

INSURANCE COVERAGE

Insurance coverage for GAS is highly variable, and often there are unclear guidelines related to the coverage of surgical procedures. Insurance coverage will be discussed in a later chapter. WPATH Version 8 states that "health care systems should provide medically necessary gender-affirming health care for transgender and gender diverse people."[8] Documentation by the health care professional of gender incongruence is sufficient to determine medically necessary gender-affirming care. Insurance coverage trends, however, have been on the increase. Of Fortune 500 companies, 91% were shown to have TGD-inclusive insurance coverage in 2022.[11]

NONGENDER BODY DYSPHORIA

BDD is defined in the *Diagnostic and Statistical Manual of Mental Disorders* (Fifth Edition) (*DSM-5*) as the preoccupation with one or more perceived defects or flaws in physical appearance that are not observable or appear slight to others.[12] During the course of the disorder, the patient performs repetitive behaviors (eg, mirror checking, excessive grooming, skin picking, reassurance seeking) or mental acts (eg, comparing his or her appearance with that of others) in response to the appearance concerns, and this preoccupation causes clinically significant distress or impairment in social, occupational, or other areas of functioning.[13] This is distinct from how the *DSM-5* characterizes gender dysphoria, which is an incongruence between one's experienced/expressed gender and assigned gender as discussed in the psychological evaluation section. No studies have assessed the prevalence of comorbid BDD and gender dysphoria in patients seeking FFS, but it has been the authors' personal experience that some patients suffer from both, which can complicate their preoperative assessment and postoperative satisfaction.[14]

Unfortunately, the most common preoccupations include skin, hair, and nose,[13] all of which are areas encountered in FFS. The suicide ideation and attempt are 80% and 25%, respectively, in BDD.[13] Most likely in a person with gender dysphoria and BDD, the postoperative outcome can be ideal; however, if there is an overlap, they may not perceive the successful nature of the surgery since the patient, "compare themselves to an impossibly ideal appearance."[13] In the authors' experience, patients who have located their ideal, for example, "nose," will be fixated on a very specific nose and may even be rigid in their ideal after being told it may not be possible. Discussing what is possible is important and should be well documented. More visits may be required until a mutual agreement is achieved, or surgery may be deferred.

During the psychological evaluation, there may exist a component of not wanting to prevent a patient from clearance for FFS and thus an additional diagnosis of BDD may be missed or underreported. Regardless, as a surgeon, it is important to be aware of this possible comorbidity and understand the significance it can have, particularly postoperatively, on the patient's satisfaction and desire for continued surgery.

EXPECTATIONS

Before pursuing any GAS, patients and their surgeon or surgeons should engage in honest discussions to better understand the patient's desired outcomes and expectations as well as any potential benefit or limitation of the planned procedure or procedures.[15] It is necessary to develop surgical plans on an individualized basis and to include the multidisciplinary team (if available) as part of this workup and discussion. The shared decision-making model should provide patients with realistic expectations for each procedure as well as for any future considered procedures. The informed consent process should focus on the permanent nature of some of the procedures and lack of long-term outcomes for some of these procedures. In addition, an informed plan for aftercare should be developed preoperatively, as a patient's expectations can continue to evolve in the perioperative period. Ultimately, the WPATH recommends that the patient and their surgeon work together to ensure the patient's expectations are realistic and achievable, and the proposed interventions are safe and technically feasible.[14]

WHEN IS THE PATIENT ACTUALLY READY FOR SURGERY

Surgeons who desire to perform GAS should complete training and have documented supervision in gender-affirming procedures. They should maintain an active practice in gender-affirming surgical procedures, be knowledgeable about gender-diverse identities and expressions, complete continuing education for GAS, and track their surgical outcomes. Once the decision has been made to pursue GAS surgery, a comprehensive perioperative and postoperative care plan should be established with the patient. A multidisciplinary team approach is recommended, especially for patients who have individualized or custom surgical requests, which the WPATH defines as follows: "(1) a procedure that alters an individual's gender expression without necessarily aiming to express an alternative, binary gender; (2) the 'non-standard' combination of well-established procedures; or (3) both."[8]

POSTSURGERY THOUGHTS

Patients undergoing gender-affirming FFS are generally satisfied with their decision to undergo surgery. In 2010, a study by Ainsworth and Spiegel[16] surveyed male-to-female transgender individuals using the FFS outcomes evaluation and the SF-36v2 quality-of-life survey. Patients who underwent gender reassignment surgery, FFS, or both were found to have an improved mental health–related quality of life compared with transgender women who had not undergone surgical intervention.

Research has been focused on quantifying the impact of gender-affirming FFS on quality of life. In a recent study, a total of 169 patients undergoing FFS were administered 11 validated, quantitative patient-reported outcomes measures before and after FFS surgery. Based on a cross-sectional assessment of psychosocial outcomes, patients receiving gender-affirming FFS reported "improved anxiety, anger, depression, positive affect, meaning and purpose, global mental health, and social isolation."[17] This has been the authors' experience at their institution as well. In addition, since the start of insurance coverage, patients who may not have been able to afford surgery out of pocket are now given the chance to have an otherwise unattainable surgery. It is hoped that insurance coverage will deter patients from having unsafe procedures from nonmedical people to avoid some of the difficulties that can occur in the future.

DISCLOSURE

The authors have no financial disclosures.

REFERENCES

1. Bueller H. Ideal Facial Relationships and Goals. Facial Plast Surg 2018;34:458–65.
2. Mommaerts MY, Moerenhout BA. Ideal proportions in full face front view, contemporary versus antique. J Craniomaxillofac Surg 2011;39(2):107–10 [published correction appears in J Craniomaxillofac Surg. 2013 Dec;41(8):705].
3. Deschamps-Braly JC. Facial Gender Confirmation Surgery: Facial Feminization Surgery and Facial Masculinization Surgery. Clin Plast Surg 2018; 45(3):323–31.
4. Callen AL, Badiee RK, Phelps A, et al. Facial Feminization Surgery: Key CT Findings for Preoperative Planning and Postoperative Evaluation. AJR Am J Roentgenol 2021;217(3):709–17.
5. Chaya B, Boczar D, Rodriguez Colon R, et al. Comparative Outcomes of Partial and Full Facial Feminization Surgery: A Retrospective Cohort Study. J Craniofac Surg 2021;32(7):2397–400.
6. Gupta N, Wulu J, Spiegel JH. Safety of Combined Facial Plastic Procedures Affecting Multiple Planes in a Single Setting in Facial Feminization for Transgender Patients. Aesthetic Plast Surg 2019;43:993–9.
7. Wang LL, Thomas WW, Friedman O. Granuloma formation secondary to silicone injection for soft-tissue augmentation in facial cosmetics: Mechanisms and literature review. Ear Nose Throat J 2018;97(1–2): E46–51.

8. World Professional Association for Transgender Health. (2022). Standards of Care for the Health of Transgender and Gender Diverse People [8th Version]. Available at: https://doi.org/10.1080/26895269.2022.2100644. Accessed January 3, 2023.

9. Meningaud JP, Benadiba L, Servant JM, et al. Depression, anxiety and quality of life: outcome 9 months after facial cosmetic surgery. J Craniomaxillofac Surg 2003;31(1):46–50.

10. Connelly PJ, Marie Freel E, Perry C, et al. Gender-Affirming Hormone Therapy, Vascular Health and Cardiovascular Disease in Transgender Adults. Hypertension 2019;74(6):1266–74 [published correction appears in Hypertension. 2020;75(4):e10].

11. Gadkaree SK, DeVore EK, Richburg K, et al. National Variation of Insurance Coverage for Gender-Affirming Facial Feminization Surgery. Facial Plast Surg Aesthet Med 2021;23(4):270–7.

12. Phillips K. Diagnostic and statistical manual of mental disorders: DSM-5. 5th edition. American Psychiatric Association; 2013. p. 242–7.

13. Fang A, Matheny NL, Wilhelm S. Body dysmorphic disorder. Psychiatr Clin North Am 2014;37(3):287–300.

14. Spiegel JH. Challenges in care of the transgender patient seeking facial feminization surgery. Facial Plast Surg Clin North Am 2008;16:233–8.

15. Brody-Camp S, Shehan JN, Spiegel JH. Approach to the Transgender Patient: Preoperative Counseling, Setting Expectations, Avoiding Potential Postoperative Pitfalls. Otolaryngol Clin North Am 2022;55:707–13.

16. Ainsworth TA, Spiegel JH. Quality of life of individuals with and without facial feminization surgery or gender reassignment surgery. Qual Life Res 2010;19(7):1019–24.

17. Caprini R, Oberoi M, Dejam D, et al. Effect of Gender-affirming Facial Feminization Surgery on Psychosocial Outcomes. Ann Surg 2022. https://doi.org/10.1097/SLA.0000000000005472.

Chondrolaryngoplasty

Katherine Nicole Vandenberg, MD[a,b], Michal Jakub Plocienniczak, MD, MSc[a,b], Jeffrey Howard Spiegel, MD[a,b,*]

KEYWORDS

- Chondrolaryngoplasty • Feminization laryngoplasty • Tracheal shave • Neck feminization
- Facial feminization

KEY POINTS

- Chondrolaryngoplasty, commonly known by the misnomer "Tracheal Shave", is a cosmetic surgical procedure designed to reduce the anterior prominence of the thyroid cartilage, the "Adam's apple".
- When performed with direct visualization of the vocal cords, a maximum reduction can be achieved safely.
- Evaluation of outcomes associated with chondrolaryngoplasty demonstrates a high rate of satisfaction and a low rate of complications.
- Chondrolaryngoplasty may be performed safely in conjunction with other facial feminization procedures.

Video content accompanies this article at http://www.facialplastic.theclinics.com.

INTRODUCTION

An understanding of laryngeal anatomy and gender differences during development is necessary to maximize outcomes and perform chondrolaryngoplasty safely. The larynx undergoes significant developmental changes and often becomes a source of gender dysphoria for transgender patients. Until puberty, the male and female laryngeal frameworks are indistinguishable from one another. After puberty, all the cartilaginous components of a male larynx become larger than their counterparts in the female larynx. The anterior-posterior dimension of the thyroid cartilage, in particular, will double in size and the entire larynx is about 20% larger in men compared with women. This size increase in part accounts for the deeper voice typical to most men. As the larynx develops from the fourth and sixth branchial arch, the laminae of the thyroid cartilage migrate and fuse anteriorly in the midline leaving a gap in the superior-most part, otherwise known as the thyroid notch. The anterior projection of this notch

or the thyroid prominence is greater in men and is often called the "Adam's apple."

Studies evaluating computed tomography images of the thyroid cartilage demonstrate significant gender-specific differences. The laminae in women are more flattened, ranging from 80° to 120°. In men, however, this angle is sharper, ranging between 63° and 90°.[1-7] Similarly, the anterior angulation of the thyroid cartilage, defined as the angle between two lines tangential to the cricothyroid membrane and the anterior face of the thyroid cartilage, is more acute (155°–167°) in men compared to women who have a more obtuse angle (168°–172°).[8] These studies demonstrate that the thyroid cartilage in men is more anteriorly rotated and the notch is sharper, creating a more prominent Adam's apple.

Chondrolaryngoplasty is more commonly, and rather inaccurately, known as a "tracheal shave", despite the fact that no intervention is performed on the trachea. It was first described by Wolfort and Parry in 1975 and further modified by Wolfort

[a] Department of Otolaryngology—Head and Neck Surgery, Division of Facial Plastic and Reconstructive Surgery, Boston University School of Medicine, 800 Harrison Avenue, BCD Building, 5th Floor, Boston, MA 02118, USA; [b] The Spiegel Center, 335 Boylston Street, Newton, MA 02459, USA
* Corresponding author. The Spiegel Center, 335 Boylston Street, Newton, MA 02459.
E-mail address: DrSpiegel@DrSpiegel.com

Facial Plast Surg Clin N Am 31 (2023) 355–361
https://doi.org/10.1016/j.fsc.2023.03.001

in 1990.[9–11] These initial approaches relied on elevating the perichondrium on the glottic surface of the thyroid cartilage to identify the thyroepiglottic ligament and thus the inferior extent of the resection. The cartilage was then reduced using a burr, however, other instruments including cautery and cold-cutting devices may also be used. Since then, the technique has been further modified to allow for more complete resection under direct visualization of the anterior commissure using a laryngeal mask and flexible laryngoscope.[12]

The absence of Adam's apple in a man is unnoticed, but the presence of Adam's apple in a woman is distinct and out of place. As a result, transgender patients seeking gender-reaffirming surgery may desire a chondrolaryngoplasty to reduce the size of their thyroid prominence. This procedure can be done safely in the operative room, oftentimes concurrently with other facial feminization procedures.

PATIENT EVALUATION

Before a surgical referral for chondrolaryngoplasty, patients must be evaluated by their medical and mental health care providers. Psychological well-being, reasonable expectations, and physical exam findings all play a role when determining who is a good candidate for chondrolaryngoplasty. For example, a patient with a slender neck and large prominent thyroid cartilage may have a more meaningful outcome than a patient with significant submental adipose tissue and a less obvious Adam's apple. On the other hand, it may be more difficult or impossible to completely remove the appearance caused by a larger thyroid cartilage on a more slender neck. The average distance between the thyroid notch and the anterior commissure is 7 mm, ranging on average between 5 and 11 mm.[13] If there is prominence of the thyroid cartilage inferior to this level, then complete removal of prominence may not be achieved without sacrificing voice quality, a tradeoff that is not acceptable and should be reinforced in patients. It is also important to realize that the degree of dysphoria does not necessarily correlate with the visibility or prominence of the thyroid notch. Additionally, sometimes the most prominent structure in the neck is not the thyroid cartilage but rather the cricoid cartilage and this must also be pointed out to patients when managing expectations as to what can be accomplished.

The position of the thyroid notch relative to the hyoid bone will determine how high the horizontal incision can be placed. Careful examination of the neck for pathology and skin quality is also paramount and if a patient has any abnormality in their

voice quality, a preoperative flexible laryngoscope exam is warranted. The incision can be hidden in the cervicomental groove, a pre-existing scar, or other prominent neck rhytids. The degree of improvement based on these anatomical considerations versus the visibility of the scar should be weighed and discussed with patients to manage their expectations and achieve a satisfactory outcome. Documentation with standardized pre- and postoperative photographs will also help show patients how much change was achieved with the procedure. Chondrolaryngoplasty may also be performed through a trans-oral approach. Here, an incision is made in the labiogingival sulcus in front of the mandibular incisors and dissection is carried into the neck through this approach. Endoscopes, additional time, and special equipment are typically required for this approach which can obviate the need for the 1–2 cm incision on the neck.

SURGICAL TECHNIQUE
Patient Position

Chondrolaryngoplasty at the senior author's center is often coupled with other facial feminization surgeries and is performed at the beginning of the case. The patient is placed in a supine position on the operative table, anesthesia is induced, and a laryngeal mask airway (LMA) is placed for ventilation. The use of an LMA is crucial to allow for direct fiberoptic visualization of the larynx during and immediately after cartilage resection.[12] The head may be flexed to permit a higher incision placement. The incision, which is approximately 1.5 cm, is horizontal and marked high in the submental neck or in the submental crease. Commonly, it can be done at the superior edge of the hyoid bone. The thyroid cartilage is also marked and the area is injected with a local anesthetic containing epinephrine (**Fig. 1**). The neck is prepared with a non-alcohol-based solution such as betadine and the patient is draped sterilely leaving the LMA exposed for the flexible bronchoscopist. Direct closed-loop communication with the anesthesiologist and maintaining an inhaled oxygen concentration below 30% is crucial to minimizing the risk of airway fire. The team should nonetheless be prepared for such a possibility with saline and appropriate safety measures available.

Surgical Steps

An incision is made sharply through the skin. Cautery use is minimized as there is no desire to eliminate subcutaneous fat which can blunt the appearance of the eventual remaining superior

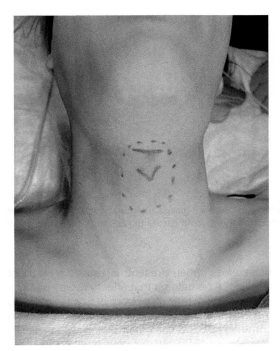

Fig. 1. Intraoperative view of the anterior neck marking the thyroid notch "V" and the superior horizontal incision "-". The area within the dotted line represents the extent of local anesthetic infiltration and undermining required for surgical exposure.

aspect of the laryngeal cartilage. Blunt vertical (sagittal) spreads are made between the strap muscles and through the midline raphe until the thyroid cartilage is encountered. The pretracheal fascia is incised and the perichondrium is lifted off the thyroid cartilage using a Cottle elevator. Exposure is accomplished using three-point retraction bilaterally and inferiorly, typically with Senn and Ragnell retractors. At this point, a

flexible bronchoscope is inserted through the LMA to visualize the larynx, ideally on a video monitor positioned where the surgeons and anesthesia team can see it. Next, under direct endoscopic visualization of the true vocal folds, a 22 gauge needle is pierced through the anterior thyroid cartilage where one anticipates an appropriate degree of resection should occur (Fig. 2). The needle must be seen to be above (superior to) the true vocal folds at the level of the thyroepiglottic ligament and above the anterior commissure. This guides the inferior extent of a safe thyroid notch reduction (Fig. 3). The fraction of inspired oxygen is confirmed to be down to 30% to allow for the safe marking of the inferior extent of the resection with cautery. The fascia on the superior edge of the thyroid cartilage is also incised with cautery. Next, the needle and flexible scope are removed, and a double action Rongeur is used to resect the thyroid cartilage starting in a just paramedian position lateral to the true midline. The midline tends to be thicker and often more calcified and is better approached later when softer lateral cartilage is removed and there is more room for maneuvering of the instruments. Care is taken to not pivot or rock the Ronguers, especially if a patient has calcified laryngeal cartilage. Fracture of the thyroid cartilage may occur and would require plating to repair if this technique is not carefully executed.[13] Ideally, the Rongeur cuts and then the forceps are minimally released while pulling in a linear fashion. This allows the cartilage to be removed while leaving any soft tissue (including the inner perichondrium) behind (Fig. 4). At the conclusion of the procedure, the flexible bronchoscope is re-inserted and the vocal folds are confirmed to be in their proper position with a sharp glottic chink. Gentle external pressure is applied to the new superior surface of the thyroid cartilage to ensure no collapse of the glottis

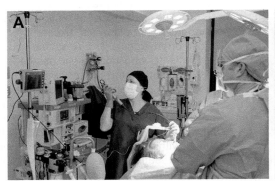
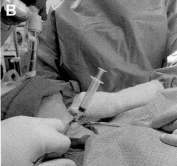

Fig. 2. (A) Effective closed-loop communication between the surgical team and the anesthetist in this case who is performing laryngoscopy through an LMA to visualize the glottis in preparation for needle insertion. (B) Anterior neck with a three-point retraction and a 22 gauge needle inserted through the thyroid cartilage.

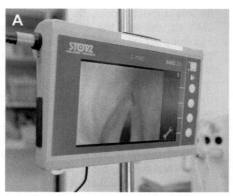
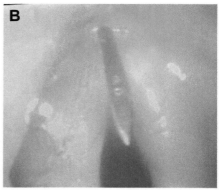

Fig. 3. (A) Video laryngoscopy during a chondrolaryngoplasty shows a 22 gauge needle above the level of the anterior commissure attachments, guiding the inferior extent of the thyroid cartilage resection. (B) Closer view of a different patient.

(Video 1). For closure, the strap muscles are re-approximated and the skin is closed in layers using 5 to 0 Vicryl and Dermabond. If other surgical procedures are to follow, at this time, the patient's airway may be secured with endotracheal intubation.

Potential Risks

The most commonly seen risks of chondrolaryngoplasty are minor and include scar from the cervical incision, unsatisfactory changes in the prominence of the thyroid notch, and temporary pain, sore throat, or hoarseness in the immediate postoperative period. The most serious risk is of permanent voice changes caused by disruption of the attachment of the vocal cords to the thyroid cartilage at the anterior commissure. Transient

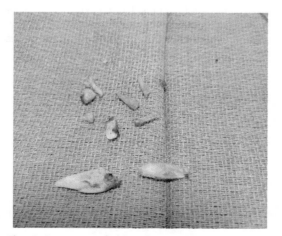

Fig. 4. Segments of thyroid cartilage removed with Rongeurs. Notice that only cartilage is removed. The soft tissue and fascia surrounding the cartilage are left in vivo.

hoarseness, when present, is usually a result of swelling. A hematoma that affects airway patency during surgery may also occur but typically would resolve quickly.[13] Another hazardous but less common risk that can occur during surgery is laryngospasm (1.5%) and a plan must be in place and communicated between the anesthesiologist and surgeon before surgery.[14]

Permanent vocal changes are a devastating risk of chondrolaryngoplasty and are a major reason why the procedure was modified so that the maximum excision of cartilage was guided by direct visualization of the larynx. Vocal phonation frequency, or pitch, behaves similarly to a piano string. Fletcher described the ideal string law in 1964, which determined that frequency is directly related to longitudinal stress, among other variables.[12] By disturbing the anterior commissure, one introduces laxity to the vocal cords and decreases longitudinal stress leading to decreased vibration frequency, and therefore, reduced pitch, significantly adversely affecting the patient's voice. This is an outcome that would not be acceptable to any woman, cis or trans. The incidence of voice changes after chondrolaryngoplasty is exceedingly rare and most often transient.[15] A systematic review of 69 patients who underwent aesthetic chondrolaryngoplasty found that no patients had permanent voice concerns post-operatively. The most common temporary complications cited in this review included odynophagia and hoarseness. Of the patients with hoarseness, 96% had resolution within 20 days and over 98% of patients reported satisfaction with the outcome.[11] Of note, permanent hoarseness has been noted by other surgeons using methods that do not involve visualization of the anterior commissure during the time of resection.

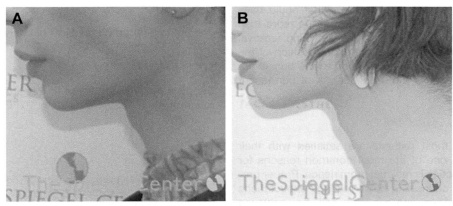

Fig. 5. (A) Pre- and (B) postoperative left lateral views of a patient with a slender neck and a larger thyroid prominence in which a smoother contour was achieved but a prominence (although smaller) is still visible.

Another retrospective survey on 48 of 198 patients who underwent aesthetic chondrolaryngoplasty found that 80% were "very" or "completely" satisfied with the appearance of their neck after surgery, while only 13% were "not at all" satisfied. The most frequent comments from less satisfied patients were of persistent prominence and size or location of the scar. No patients had permanent voice changes. All of these patients underwent chondrolaryngoplasty with direct visualization of the true vocal folds during and immediately after the procedure.[15] It is important to counsel patients that the extent of the Adam's apple resection is limited by the attachment of the vocal folds and that function must not be jeopardized over aesthetic results.

POST-OPERATIVE CARE

Care required by patients after a chondrolaryngoplasty is minimal. A majority of these cases are combined with other facial feminization procedures and these other procedures dictate the perioperative care. Pain is typically minimal and may include a sore throat from intubation. As the incision is closed with Dermabond, no incision care is needed. Patients are typically discharged home the same day from the post-anesthesia care unit.

ALTERNATIVE APPROACHES

One drawback of this traditional approach is the potential for an unsightly scar. Although scar revision and resurfacing techniques largely mitigate these potential complications, recent publications have begun to emerge describing trans-oral trans-vestibular approaches that obviate the need for a cervical incision. In these cases, the approach is similar to a trans-vestibular endoscopic thyroidectomy and once the thyroid prominence is encountered, a burr is used to shave down the notch until the desired aesthetic outcome is achieved. Due to the need for straight instruments, a bulky LMA is not possible, therefore, direct visualization of the true vocal cords is limited during the procedure. Also, one can imagine how difficult it may be to remove the lateral lamina of the thyroid notch. Although a scar can be avoided, there is a risk of

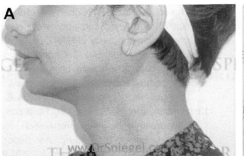

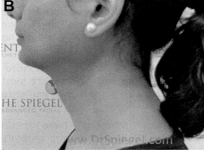

Fig. 6. (A) Pre- and (B) postoperative left lateral views of a patient with anatomy that allowed for maximal resection of the thyroid cartilage resulting in a completely smooth anterior neck.

leaving behind thyroid cartilage that could have otherwise been removed or removing more than should have been removed. With blind removal of the thyroid cartilage, the exact position of the anterior commissure in relation to the burr is not known and may increase the risk of permanent voice injury.[16–18]

CLINICAL OUTCOMES

Although most patients are satisfied with their outcome, one of the most common reasons for dissatisfaction is residual prominence. Proper preoperative counseling helps manage expectations and a softer contour can still be achieved (**Fig. 5**). Other patients may have anatomy that allows for maximum reduction in the thyroid cartilage creating a smooth anterior neck without shadowing from the thyroid notch (**Fig. 6**).

SUMMARY

Chondrolaryngoplasty is a safe and effective surgical procedure that reduces the prominence of the thyroid notch. It is most commonly performed on transgender (man to woman) patients with gender dysphoria and may be performed alone or in combination with other facial feminization procedures. Overall, patients are very satisfied with the outcomes of chondrolaryngoplasty and risks are low. Although scarless methods have been described, there is a tradeoff and direct visual guidance is made more difficult if not impossible.

CLINICS CARE POINTS

- Chondrolaryngoplasty is a safe and effective procedure for removing the prominence of the thyroid cartilage.
- Preoperative evaluation and management of expectations are crucial to patient satisfaction.
- Direct visualization of the anterior commissure using a laryngeal airway and flexible bronchoscope allows surgeons to remove most of the cartilage without jeopardizing vocal quality.
- Postoperative complications from chondrolaryngoplasty are rare and patients are most often dissatisfied with a residual prominence or scar.
- Though scarless methods have been described, they are limited by the inability to guide maximum resection through direct visualization of the anterior commissure.

DISCLOSURE

The authors report no conflicts of interest.

SUPPLEMENTARY DATA

Supplementary data related to this article can be found online at https://doi.org/10.1016/j.fsc.2023.03.001.

REFERENCES

1. Ajmani M. A metrical study of the laryngeal skeleton in adult Nigerians. J Anat 1990;171:187.
2. Ajmani M, Jain S, Saxena S. A metrical study of laryngeal cartilages and their ossification. Anat Anz 1980;148(1):42–8.
3. Sagiv D, Eyal A, Mansour J, et al. Novel anatomic characteristics of the laryngeal framework: a computed tomography evaluation. Otolaryngol Neck Surg 2016;154(4):674–8.
4. Eckel HE, Sprinzl GM, Koebke J, et al. Morphology of the human larynx during the first five years of life studied on whole organ serial sections. Ann Otol Rhinol Laryngol 1999;108(3):232–8.
5. Eckel HE, Sittel C. Morphometry of the larynx in horizontal sections. Am J Otolaryngol 1995;16(1):40–8.
6. Kovač T, Popović B, Marjanović K, et al. Morphometric characteristics of thyroid cartilage in people of Eastern Croatia. Coll Antropol 2010;34(3):1069–73.
7. Sprinzl GM, Eckel HE, Sittel C, et al. Morphometric measurements of the cartilaginous larynx: an anatomic correlate of laryngeal surgery. Head Neck J Sci Spec Head Neck 1999;21(8):743–50.
8. Glikson E, Sagiv D, Eyal A, et al. The anatomical evolution of the thyroid cartilage from childhood to adulthood: A computed tomography evaluation. Laryngoscope 2017;127(10):E354–8.
9. WOLFORT FG, PARRY RG. Laryngeal chondroplasty for appearance. Plast Reconstr Surg 1975;56(4):371–4.
10. Wolfort FG, Dejerine ES, Ramos DJ, et al. Chondrolaryngoplasty for appearance. Plast Reconstr Surg 1990;86(3):464–9.
11. Therattil PJ, Hazim NY, Cohen WA, et al. Esthetic reduction of the thyroid cartilage: a systematic review of chondrolaryngoplasty. JPRAS Open 2019;22:27–32.
12. Spiegel JH, Rodriguez G. Chondrolaryngoplasty under general anesthesia using a flexible fiberoptic laryngoscope and laryngeal mask airway. Arch Otolaryngol Neck Surg 2008;134(7):704–8.
13. Hassanzadeh T, Spiegel JH. Rare complications in chondrolaryngoplasty: preparation for safe outcomes. Facial Plast Surg Aesthetic Med 2022. https://doi.org/10.1089/fpsam.2022.0240.
14. Therattil PJ, Hazim NY, Cohen WA, et al. Esthetic reduction of the thyroid cartilage: a systematic

review of chondrolaryngoplasty. JPRAS Open 2019;
22:27–32.

15. Cohen MB, Insalaco LF, Tonn CR, et al. Patient
satisfaction after aesthetic chondrolaryngoplasty.
Plast Reconstr Surg Glob Open 2018;6(10):
e1877.

16. Khafif A, Shoffel-Havakuk H, Yaish I, et al. Scarless
neck feminization: transoral transvestibular approach

chondrolaryngoplasty. Facial Plast Surg Aesthetic
Med 2020;22(3):172–80.

17. Chung J, Purnell P, Anderson S, et al. Transoral chondrolaryngoplasty: scarless reduction of the Adam's
apple. OTO Open 2020;4(3). 2473974X20938299.

18. Verhasselt M, Cavelier G, Horoi M, et al. Chondrolaryngoplasty for transgender patients: feasibility of a
scar-free approach. Eur Arch Oto-Rhino-Laryngol
2020;277:2381–4.

Forehead Contouring

Nikita Gupta, MD*, Carly Clark, MD

KEYWORDS

- Forehead contouring • Upper third of face • Facial feminization • Gender affirmation facial surgery

KEY POINTS

- A thorough facial analysis is required from both the patient and the surgeon to determine areas of concern and appropriate management is indicated based on the patient's anatomy.
- The majority of patients that desire contouring will require an open surgical approach including cranioplasty with frontal sinus anterior table setback.
- Although facial feminization procedures are generally well tolerated, risks for forehead contouring procedures include infection, hematoma formation, hair loss, paresthesia, and scarring.
- Facial feminization surgery is an important and effective treatment of gender dysphoria and has been shown to improve quality of life outcomes in transgender women.

INTRODUCTION

The goal of facial feminization procedures is to alter facial features in order for observers to identify a person as a woman. This is frequently utilized as a part of gender-affirming facial surgery for those identifying as trans-feminine, but the principles can also be applied to cis women desiring features considered more classically feminine. The upper third of the face has been shown to have an important effect on gendering patients. Forehead contouring modifying a masculine face to a more feminine form is most likely to affect the gender assessment of an individual's face.[1]

BACKGROUND

Dr Douglas Ousterhout first described specific skeletal characteristics that contribute to the identification of an individual as man or woman in 1987.[2] After analyzing hundreds of cadaver skulls and patients, he created a classification system for forehead contouring that consists of three groups. He used the projection of supraorbital rims, the degree of bossing, and the thickness of bone over the frontal sinus to categorize each patient's degree of deformity and the appropriate intervention.

This system formed an important basis to help examine exactly what features can be targeted to help create a feminine appearance. After establishing the patient's areas of concern, we can provide guidance on addressing the face as a whole unit to achieve the most successful results. Forehead contouring serves as one strategy to create a more feminine appearance.

The upper third of the face is a key determinant of femininity and gender. Both bony protuberances and soft tissue features are components of this assessment. Masculine features include a prominent glabella and supraorbital ridges, deep-set orbits, eyebrow shape and position, and a high, M-shaped hairline. Feminizing these features has the greatest effect on viewers' impressions of gender.

In studies of observers rating gender based on facial images with altered features, Spiegel demonstrated that the upper third of the face is the most significant area for determining gender. He showed there is a strong association between femininity and attractiveness specifically attributed to the upper third of the face and the interplay of the glabellar prominence, eyebrow shape and position, and hairline shape and position.[1] This has additionally been confirmed via 3D morphology facial assessment

University of Kentucky Otolaryngology- Head and Neck Surgery, Division of Facial Plastic and Reconstructive Surgery, 740 South Limestone, E305, Lexington, KY 40536, USA
* Corresponding author.
E-mail address: Nikita.gupta@uky.edu

Facial Plast Surg Clin N Am 31 (2023) 363–370
https://doi.org/10.1016/j.fsc.2023.03.003
1064-7406/23/© 2023 Elsevier Inc. All rights reserved.

quantifying the effect of facial size and shape in the forehead and other facial regions.[3] Studies of gender recognition showed a 96% ability to correctly identify gender by face alone even when stripped of secondary characteristics such as hairstyle, facial hair pattern, cosmetics, and jewelry.[4] Femininity and attractiveness are linked in facial assessment as increasing feminization of faces leads to higher ratings of attractiveness.

Current practice is based on literature regarding observers' perceptions of femininity. However, patients have different motivations for undergoing surgery that are not limited to these external observer perceptions. Gender-affirming facial surgery has been shown to have positive effects on mental health-related quality of life.[5,6] Ultimately, surgical care is determined on an individual basis depending on the concerns/dysphoria of the patient and guidance by the surgeon.

Clinical Relevance

Transgender patients who desire surgery frequently meet the criteria for gender dysphoria. The diagnosis requires a strong and persistent cross-gender identification, discomfort with the patient's assigned sex and its associated role, and the absence of a physical intersex condition.[5] Without intervention, including gender affirmation surgery and/or facial feminization, patients can suffer from depression and anxiety. When comparing transgender women who underwent facial feminization surgery (FFS) to those who have not, those with intervention are shown to have a higher mental health-related quality of life scores.[5] Further, patients report improvements in self-perception and public perception following FFS, which may alleviate symptoms of gender dysphoria.[6]

Evaluation

- Facial Analysis of the Upper Third of the Face
  An individualized approach to each patient is key to achieving the most appropriate surgical outcome. Facial analysis of the upper third of the face helps identify masculine features to address with each patient. Age and timing of beginning hormone therapy are factors in this analysis as well.
  - Hairline–Assess hairline shape, position, hair quality, and density as well as the forehead/scalp skin laxity
    - Temporal recession with 'M'-shaped hairline in men[7]
  - Forehead–Assess bony protuberances
    - Remember to consider projection of forehead in relation to nose, nasofrontal angle

- Forehead contouring often performed in conjunction with other procedures
- Improved patient satisfaction with rhinoplasty when performed in conjunction with forehead contouring[8]
  - Glabellar bossing
    - Often related to increased aeration of the frontal sinus though could be related to thin anterior table bone with minimal aeration[2,9]
  - Supraorbital bossing
    - Men often have prominent supraorbital ridges and/or larger frontal sinuses[7]
    - Ensure that there is true supraorbital bossing rather than depressed frontal bone
  - Consider treating frontal bone depression with augmentation rather than supraorbital contouring
    - Slope of forehead
      - Smoother and sloping forehead in women compared to flat forehead in men[8]
    - Transition between frontal and nasal compartments
- Acute transition in men[8] with average angle of 130° versus 134° in women[7]
  - Temples and soft tissue
    - Temporal hollowing in men compared to women[10]
  - Brows–Evaluate position in relation to orbital rim, shape, and arch pattern
    - Arched brows that sit above the orbital rim appear more feminine[11]
  - Eyelids–Evaluate shape, hooding, excess skin, rhytids
- Structural considerations
  - Forehead shape classification system defined by Dr Douglas Ousterhout[2,10]
    - Group I (8%–9%): Mild to moderate anterior projection of the supraorbital rims, thick frontal bone, and/or absence of frontal sinus
      - Thick frontal bone amenable to burring along, without entering frontal sinus
    - Group II (8%–9%): Mild to moderate anterior projection of the supraorbital rims with thin frontal bone with normal-sized frontal sinus
      - These patients often have an area of concavity superior to the supraorbital rim requiring augmentation
    - Group III (83%): Extensive supraorbital anterior projection not amenable to contouring without entering the frontal sinus
      - Anterior table of the frontal sinus requires osteotomy with setback to achieve adequate contouring

o Frontal sinus anatomy
- Aplastic and/or asymmetric size of frontal sinuses[7]
- Sinuses extend more laterally with more forward projection in men than women[12] (**Fig. 1**)
- Anterior table thickness

DISCUSSION

The forehead, including glabellar and supraorbital bossing, hairline shape and position, and eyebrow position, has a significant impact on observers determining the gender of a person. Procedures that can address these features include

- Cranioplasty with frontal sinus anterior table setback
  - o Most commonly performed/indicated procedure
  - o Required for patients with thin anterior table and/or severe frontal bossing (Ousterhout Group III)
  - o Steps:
    - Anterior table of frontal sinus is outlined and then removed (**Fig. 2**)
      - Various techniques for identifying location of sinus include
        - o Measurements from pre-operative imaging including computed tomography (CT) or x-ray
        - o Intraoperative frontal sinus illumination[13]
        - o 3D printed cutting guide[14]
    - Contour and reduce intersinus septum
    - Evaluate sinus mucosa and patency of frontal sinus outflow tract
    - Flatten bone flap along outer and inner surfaces to create a smooth surface
    - Reposition the bony plate with plates and screws (**Figs. 3 and 4**)
    - Autologous bone pate used to fill in defects and help with healing
- Supraorbital contouring
  - o Burring of excess bone laterally to achieve aesthetic goals
  - o Take care to achieve symmetry on both sides
  - o Dissect in a deep to plane laterally to avoid the frontal branch of the facial nerve injury[13]
- Brow lift
  - o Affects height and morphology of the eyebrows
  - o Soft tissue excision to achieve this goal via the same incision chosen for approach to the bony forehead

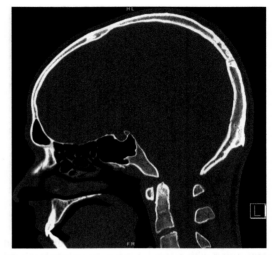

Fig. 1. Sagittal view of transwoman before forehead contouring procedure demonstrates pneumatization and forward projection of frontal sinus.

  - o May include additional suspension via suture anchors or bony channels and suture suspension[10]
- Hairline advancement
  - o Lower hairline is more feminine
  - o Typically achieved using pretrichial incision and posterior advancement of the scalp
  - o Galeotomies may be utilized for more scalp mobility

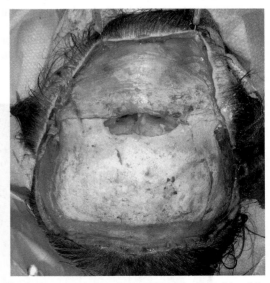

Fig. 2. Intraoperative view of the anterior table of the frontal sinus removed. Intersinus septum must be reduced to replace the contoured anterior table plate. Supraorbital bossing can be contoured directly using a drill.

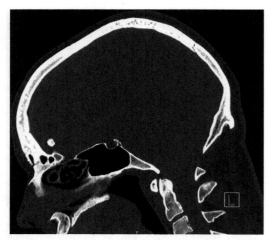

Fig. 3. Sagittal view post-operatively after forehead contouring with osteoplastic flap to reduce forehead projection.

- Lateral advancement to round M-shaped hairline (excise bitemporal recessions)[15]
- Forehead augmentation
  - Consider augmentation rather than contouring if forehead protrusion is relative to isolated supraorbital bossing without frontal bone thickening (Group II)
  - Methods include
    - Silicone implants
      - Can create custom implants based on imaging that contour exactly as desired
      - Flexible, can be placed through small scalp incisions behind the frontal hairline
        - One method is to roll the implant for insertion and then unfold once inside the implant pocket[12]

- Consider superior screw placement for fixation of the implant to avoid inferior or lateral displacement
- There is a risk of foreign body reaction or implant migration/malposition
- Tissue contraction post-operatively can reveal minor surface irregularities or result in overcorrection[12]
- Bone cement
  - Self-curing plastic polymer that can be molded and set in the bony defect
  - Materials include polymethyl methacrylate (PMMA) and hydroxyapatite (HA)
  - Cement must be placed medial to temporal fascia because it becomes unstable when placed onto fascia[12]
  - For PMMA, there is a higher risk of infection
    - Should not use PMMA at the same time as osteotomies or any entrance into the sinus due to risk of bacterial seeding from sinuses[2]
    - In contrast, HA is osteoconductive, with gradual replacement of the material with bone, making it resistant to infection[16]
  - There are case reports of patients with an inflammatory immunologic reaction to HA resulting in skin erosion and exposure to the underlying material[16]

Pre-Operative Considerations

- Imaging
  - Typically maxillofacial CT
  - Provides data regarding the frontal sinus, including anterior table thickness, extent of sinus boundaries along the forehead

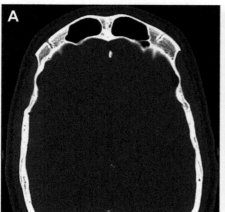
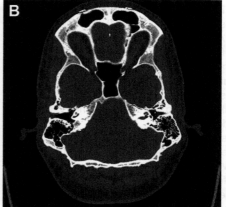

Fig. 4. Coronal views of pre-operative (*A*) and post-operative (*B*) frontal sinus. Images appear at different levels due to a change in patient positioning.

- Confirms Ousterhout classification and appropriate surgical plan
  - Rule out sinusitis, mucocele, previous trauma/surgery, or other potential pathology affecting outcomes
  - Not required and many surgeons do not perform, may be an additional cost to the patient

Surgical Techniques

- A large incision is required when performing a traditional cranioplasty. Dissection of the forehead flap should extend to the nasofrontal and orbitofrontal sutures lines, and approximately 1 cm into the orbit to allow adequate exposure of the supraorbital rim.[17]
  - Considerations when determining incision location include
    - Bicoronal
      - Entire incision is made within the hair through the periosteum to approach the bony architecture
      - Pros: Incision is hidden in the hair
      - Cons: Can cause hypesthesia, widened scar, hair loss along incision, if concurrent brow lift is desired, it is important to discuss that the patient's hairline will rise as well
    - Pretrichial
      - Centrally, the incision is along the hairline, laterally within the hair as in the bicoronal
      - Can be used to lower and reshape the hairline with advancement flaps for the bitemporal recessions[15]
      - Beveled incision in irregular pattern to mimic natural hairline to reduce visibility
      - Pros: Can perform hairline advancement and brow lift if desired
      - Cons: Visible scar, more so during the healing process

Complications

- Each procedure has inherent complications. These include
  - Hematoma–Fluid collections can occur under the scalp flap
    - Monitor closely post-operatively and drain as needed. This can be done via needle drainage or by removing a staple.
    - Can prevent with compression dressings post-operatively. Some surgeons utilize drains for prevention.

- Scarring –Bicoronal incisions can be hidden, but scarring will occur at pretrichial incision sites.
  - Patients should be counseled about scar care, particularly with respect to hairline incisions.
  - Care should be taken with any activity that can put tension on the wound such as hair brushing on putting on hats/hair pieces after sutures/staples have been removed.
  - Scalp incisions often have more crusting, requiring more post-operative care than other sites.
  - Hair loss–Telogen effluvium (shock hair loss) can occur when operating on the scalp. Additionally, hair loss may occur along the hairline incision. Patients should be counseled to manage expectations.
    - Use of feminizing hormones stabilizes the hair follicles and prevents continued androgen-related hair loss[17]
    - Bevel incisions to prevent damage to hair follicles and allow hair to grow through the scar.
    - Take care with electrocautery to protect hair follicles.
  - Cerebrospinal fluid leak–This is a possibility when working with forehead contouring but rare.
    - May occur if frontal sinus osteotomy is too high with damage to the posterior table of the frontal sinus and violation of the dura[10]
    - Angle the saw blade at 45° when removing the anterior table to prevent contact with posterior table[18]
    - Thorough inspection of frontal sinus mucosa before replacing the anterior table plate
  - Surgical emphysema–Introduction of air into the frontal sinus can occur post-operatively and potentially lead to infection[7]
    - Instruct patients to follow sinus precautions including not blowing the nose, avoid straining, and sneeze with the mouth open
  - Numbness–Decreased sensation is expected posterior to coronal/pretrichial incisions
    - Care is taken not to damage the supraorbital and facial nerves during dissection.
    - Scalp sensation may take months to return, and care should be taken when styling hair using heat to prevent burns.
  - Swelling–Typical post-operative swelling occurs at all operative sites. It is important

to counsel patients regarding assessing results during recovery.

- ○ Infection–As with any surgery, infection is a risk. This may occur in the form of a wound infection, infected hematoma, or infected implant/hardware.
  - Perioperative antibiotics and close postoperative monitoring are important in prevention and early detection to allow for appropriate treatment.
  - Use of post-operative antibiotics is at the discretion of the surgeon.
  - Post-operative sinusitis is possible, though the incidence of post-operative sinusitis appears to be consistent with that of the general population.
- No significant difference in post-operative Sinonasal Outcome Test (SNOT)-22 scores when comparing post-operative scores of patients undergoing forehead cranioplasty to a large non-symptomatic control population.[19]
  - ○ Mucocele–Any trauma to the frontal sinus mucosa may result in the formation of a delayed mucocele.
    - When looking at patients with facial trauma, mucocele formation occurs anywhere from 1 to 35 years following the inciting event with 50% of cases during the first 16 years.[19]
  - ○ Need for revision–Any facial procedure carries a risk of revision in the future, and it is important to discuss this with each patient. Asymmetry, scarring, or results that are not in line with expectations may result in requests for revision.
    - It is important to counsel patients about waiting for swelling to subside and scars to heal before consideration of further surgery.

FUTURE DIRECTIONS

- Minimally invasive techniques
  - ○ Eggshell technique described by Villepelet[11]
    - Patients with existing thin anterior wall of frontal sinus or thinned wall with burring intraoperatively
    - Use a swab, mallet, or finger to cave in the anterior wall while preserving mucosa of the frontal sinus
    - No placement of screws or plates required
  - ○ Endoscopic technique described by Guyuron[9]
    - Appropriate patient selection is required, including patients with mild frontal

bossing and thick anterior table of the frontal sinus assessed on pre-operative imaging
    - Only requires three small incisions, each about 1.5 cm in length
    - Must have adequate anterior frontal sinus wall thickness with mild frontal bossing amenable to contouring with burr and shaver (Group I or II)
- Three-dimensional planning/ virtual surgical planning
  - ○ Uses CT imaging to model the desired contour and print patient-specific cutting guides
    - Although pre-operative imaging is not routinely performed for forehead contouring, review of imaging in this case also allows for the identification of anatomic anomalies that alter the surgical technique
  - ○ Placement of the guide on the patient's forehead allows the surgeon to make cuts along pre-planned lines for frontal sinus and supraorbital rim osteotomies[14]
  - ○ Utilized in head and neck cancer with microvascular reconstruction, pediatric craniofacial reconstruction which has been shown to reduce operative time[14]
  - ○ Allows novice surgeons to develop experience with precise guidance
    - Planning guide maintains symmetry within millimeters
    - Known and demonstrated cranial depth prevents intracranial injury
  - ○ Helpful in complex or revision cases with limited surface anatomy
  - ○ Must consider the additional cost and time associated, requires extra planning/preparation before procedure as well as lead time to receive the guides

SUMMARY

The upper third of the face has been shown to have an important effect on gendering patients. Forehead contouring modifying a masculine face to a more feminine form is most likely to affect gender assessment of an individual's face (Fig. 5). Contouring involves techniques such as forehead reduction or augmentation and orbital contouring and is done in conjunction with soft tissue procedures to elevate the eyebrows and reshape the hairline. Traditionally, surgeons have utilized an open surgical technique, which is still required for significant frontal bossing, though newer innovations such as endoscopic procedures and custom implants provide an alternative

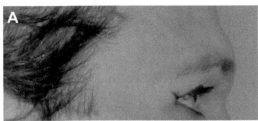
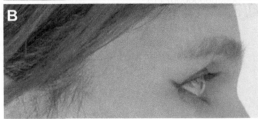

Fig. 5. Lateral view pre-operative (*A*) and post-operative (*B*) forehead contouring. (*Courtesy of* Dr Jeffrey Spiegel.)

for patients with mild defects. Forehead contouring procedures are generally well tolerated with minimal side effects reported despite the proximity to the frontal sinus and cranial vault.

CLINICS CARE POINTS

- When feasible, address multiple areas of concern while under anesthesia with the same incision.
- Frontal sinuses are asymmetrical and extend farther laterally in men than women.
- Always examine the integrity of the frontal sinus mucosa and frontal sinus outflow tract before replacing the bone flap in a cranioplasty. Ensure that there are no dural defects and that the outflow tract is patent to prevent post-operative complications.
- Take care to avoid the frontal branch of the facial nerve by dissecting deep into the temporalis fascia. Identify and protect the supraorbital nerves with any forehead flap.
- Scalp sensation may take months to return, and care should be taken when styling hair using heat to prevent burns.

DISCLOSURE

The authors have no relevant commercial or financial interests to disclose.

REFERENCES

1. Spiegel JH. Facial determinants of female gender and feminizing forehead cranioplasty. Laryngoscope 2011;121(2):250–61.
2. Ousterhout DK. Feminization of the forehead: contour changing to improve female aesthetics. Plast Reconstr Surg 1987;79(5):701–13.
3. Bannister JJ, Juszczak H, Aponte JD, et al. Sex Differences in Adult Facial Three-Dimensional Morphology: Application to Gender-Affirming Facial Surgery. Facial Plast Surg Aesthet Med 2022;24(S2):S24–30. https://doi.org/10.1089/fpsam.2021.0301.
4. Bruce V, Burton AM, Hanna E, et al. Sex discrimination: how do we tell the difference between male and female faces? Perception 1993;22(2):131–52. https://doi.org/10.1068/p220131.
5. Ainsworth TA, Spiegel JH. Quality of life of individuals with and without facial feminization surgery or gender reassignment surgery. Qual Life Res 2010;19(7):1019–24. https://doi.org/10.1007/s11136-010-9668-7.
6. Chou DW, Bruss D, Tejani N, et al. Quality of Life Outcomes After Facial Feminization Surgery. Facial Plast Surg Aesthet Med 2022;24(S2):S44–6. https://doi.org/10.1089/fpsam.2021.0373.
7. Altman K. Forehead reduction and orbital contouring in facial feminisation surgery for transgender females. Br J Oral Maxillofac Surg 2018;56(3):192–7. https://doi.org/10.1016/j.bjoms.2018.01.009.
8. Demirel O. Forehead Contouring as an Adjunct to Rhinoplasty: Evaluation of the Effect on Facial Appearance, Personal Traits and Patient Satisfaction. Aesthetic Plast Surg 2021;45(5):2257–66. https://doi.org/10.1007/s00266-021-02236-0.
9. Guyuron B, Lee M, Larson K, et al. Endoscopic correction of frontal bossing. Plast Reconstr Surg 2013;131(3):388e–93e. https://doi.org/10.1097/PRS.0b013e31827cf6ef.
10. Dang BN, Hu AC, Bertrand AA, et al. Evaluation and treatment of facial feminization surgery: part I. forehead, orbits, eyebrows, eyes, and nose. Arch Plast Surg. Sep 2021;48(5):503–10. https://doi.org/10.5999/aps.2021.00199.
11. Villepelet A, Jafari A, Baujat B. Fronto-orbital feminization technique. A surgical strategy using fronto-orbital burring with or without eggshell technique to optimize the risk/benefit ratio. Eur Ann Otorhinolaryngol Head Neck Dis 2018;135(5):353–6. https://doi.org/10.1016/j.anorl.2018.04.007.
12. Eppley BL. Forehead/Brow Reduction or Augmentation with Custom Implants for Enhanced Facial Profileplasty. Facial Plast Surg 2019;35(5):430–45. https://doi.org/10.1055/s-0039-1697962.
13. Gilde JE, Shih CW, Kleinberger AJ. Frontal Sinus Transillumination in Cranioplasty for Facial Feminization Surgery. JAMA Facial Plast Surg 2019;21(6):566–7. https://doi.org/10.1001/jamafacial.2019.0606.

14. Alperovich M. Commentary: Virtual Surgical Planning and Patient-Specific Implants in Facial Feminization Surgery. Facial Plast Surg Aesthet Med 2022;24(S2):S20–3. https://doi.org/10.1089/fpsam.2022.0302.

15. Garcia-Rodriguez L, Thain LM, Spiegel JH. Scalp advancement for transgender women: Closing the gap. Laryngoscope. Jun 2020;130(6):1431–5. https://doi.org/10.1002/lary.28370.

16. Hoenig JF. Frontal bone remodeling for gender reassignment of the male forehead: a gender-reassignment surgery. Aesthetic Plast Surg 2011; 35(6):1043–9. https://doi.org/10.1007/s00266-011-9731-y.

17. Spiegel JH. Gender affirming and aesthetic cranioplasty: what's new? Curr Opin Otolaryngol Head Neck Surg 2020;28(4):201–5. https://doi.org/10.1097/MOO.0000000000000640.

18. Eisemann BS, Wilson SC, Ramly EP, et al. Technical Pearls in Frontal and Periorbital Bone Contouring in Gender-Affirmation Surgery. Plast Reconstr Surg 2020;146(3):326e–9e. https://doi.org/10.1097/PRS.0000000000007113.

19. Basa K, Lee A, Shehan JN, et al. Frontal Bone Cranioplasty for Facial Feminization: Long-Term Follow-Up of Postoperative Sinonasal Symptoms. Facial Plast Surg Aesthet Med 2021. https://doi.org/10.1089/fpsam.2021.0037.

Getting to Yes
Navigating the Insurance Gauntlet

Jacob E. Kuperstock, MD

KEYWORDS

- Facial feminization • Transgender • Gender affirming • Insurance • Surgery

KEY POINTS

- Insurance carriers have varying policies on gender-affirming treatment medical necessity, coverage, and current procedural terminology (CPT) coding.
- Letters of medical necessity/support are often required.
- There is not a defined set of CPT codes to represent facial feminization surgery. Use of unlisted CPT codes is common.
- Employer-based insurance contracts/offerings can differ for gender-affirming surgery coverage even within the same insurer carrier network.
- Single case agreements/letters of agreement are highly recommended.

INTRODUCTION

Insurance coverage of gender-affirming surgeries including facial and vocal feminization surgery remains a challenge for many patients, physicians, and practice administrators. These challenges range from disparities in coverage for commercial versus public insurance carriers, in-network versus out-of-network benefits, preauthorization struggles, and the lack of standard coverage policies.[1-6] However, insurance coverage of gender-affirming procedures has been increasing across multiple insurance carriers in the United States.[5,7] This article aims to describe the insurance coverage and approval challenges related to facial feminization surgery (FFS) and to provide guidance for surgeons and their practice administrators on how to obtain successful preauthorization/predetermination, single case agreements, and proper claim adjudication.

CONSULTATION AND DOCUMENTATION

As with any initial patient evaluation, a complete history and physical is essential to understanding the concerns of a patient seeking FFS. Gender identity disorders have a defined ICD-10 code set of F64.X (F64.0 – F64.9).[8] Establishing and/or confirming these diagnoses for a consulting patient is critical for the consideration of gender-affirming surgery. However, a facial feminization surgeon should not be the only physician evaluating or treating a transgender patient for gender dysphoria. Mental health experts and hormone therapy prescribers should be actively treating and following-up with patients considering gender-affirming surgeries.[9]

Insurance carriers typically require letters of support/medical necessity from these practitioners and combining letters of support with good clinical documentation can lead to insurance approval success.[10-12] Having these letters of support is crucial for successful insurance coverage of FFS although there are varying policies and number of letters of support required. It is important to note that the most recent edition of the World Professional Association for Transgender Health (WPATH) Standards of Care recommends only 1 letter of support for patients planning to undergo gender-affirming surgery but this recommendation does not align with many insurance policies.[9]

Clinical documentation specifically for an FFS consultation should include whether a patient has been diagnosed with gender dysphoria,

Prior publication: This article has not been previously presented or submitted for publication.
Department of Facial Plastic and Reconstructive Surgery, Otolaryngology Associates, PC, 3801 University Drive, Suite 100, Fairfax, VA 22030, USA
E-mail address: jkuperstock@entmds.net

Facial Plast Surg Clin N Am 31 (2023) 371–374
https://doi.org/10.1016/j.fsc.2023.03.005

hormone therapy treatment (type and duration should be included), in addition to areas of the head, neck, and face that accentuate their gender dysphoria. These factors should be included in addition to the patient's past medical/surgical history (make sure to include earlier gender-affirming procedures), psychiatric history, and the physical examination. Although outside the scope of this article, there are specific facial features and structures that lead to masculine visual cues. These facial components should be included in the physical examination in addition to photodocumentation to provide congruent evidence of masculine facial features that can be surgically altered leading to feminine visual cues. Changing the craniofacial anatomy to demonstrate feminine qualities can help treat a patient's gender dysphoria and allow transgender patients to live as their genuine self. This is the basis of gender-affirming medical necessity, insurance coverage, and subsequent surgical treatment.

CONFIRMING BENEFITS AND PREAUTHORIZATION

Two terms that any FFS surgeon and their administrative team should understand is (1) preauthorization and (2) predetermination. These are two separate processes in the insurance coverage cycle. Preauthorization is a process by which medical necessity is determined for a proposed surgical or medical treatment.[13] However, not all insurance policies require preauthorization before a surgery and preauthorization also does not guarantee benefits, coverage, or payment. This is often confusing and misleading by many insurance carriers. It would seem prudent for any gender-affirming surgeon to have a patient's insurer preoperatively agree that gender-affirming services are medically necessary before rendering those services; yet some insurance policies do not have a guaranteed mechanism for preauthorization review. For example, some preferred provider organization policies do not require preauthorization for outpatient services. As such, sometimes discussing individual cases with a local insurer representative is needed to adequately obtain preauthorization for FFS.

In addition, predetermination is also not required by most insurance carriers and is considered an additional administrative step/privilege instead of requirement. Predetermination is a process where the proposed surgical or medical treatment is evaluated to see if it is included in a patient's insurance benefit plan.[14] For example, there are unfortunate situations where preauthorization has been submitted and successfully documented but benefits/coverage were not verified and/or documentation of verification was not obtained. A surgeon may move forward with the surgical procedure given the successful preauthorization but on claim adjudication, the claim is either partially or fully denied due to the lack of benefit coverage for some or all of the current procedural terminology (CPT) codes submitted. Claim adjudication is especially troublesome with unlisted procedure codes because there is no definitive procedure description or contracted rate available for these CPT codes. This is a common example where medical necessity is established with successful preauthorization despite the patient not having benefit coverage for the services. An insurer can provide preauthorization for noncovered services since medical necessity determination is separate from benefit coverage analysis. To many gender-affirming surgeons, this nuance within the insurance approval process is not logical. It is the author's opinion that this loophole should not be allowed and that insurers should not be able to provide preauthorization for facial feminization or any other medically necessary procedure, if it is not a covered benefit under the patient's insurance plan. As such, it is imperative for any surgeon willing to work with insurance to cover FFS to complete both preauthorization and predetermination.

IN-NETWORK AND OUT-OF-NETWORK STATUS/SINGLE CASE AGREEMENTS

Contracts between surgeons/practices and insurers establish varying coverage relationships for patients to access. If a contract does not exist between a surgeon and an insurance carrier, then the surgeon is considered out-of-network. Many surgeons elect for this strategy as negotiating with insurance carriers can be difficult, and time consuming. If there is an active agreement between the 2 parties, then they are considered in-network. This in-network versus out-of-network status influences the financial liability a patient might face when undergoing FFS, and the practice's reimbursement. The financial impact for both a practice and patient is also specific to a patient's insurance policy since deductible, coinsurance, and out-of-pocket maximums can all vary.

To help protect the financial liability to a facial feminization surgeon and patient, a single case agreement (also known as a letter of agreement) is highly recommended before moving forward with surgery. These are often difficult to obtain but a single case agreement establishes covered benefits for FFS including what CPT codes are being completed and their subsequent agreed on reimbursement. This is mandatory for out-of-network surgeons and is still recommended for in-network surgeons. Obtaining a single case agreement reduces but does not eliminate the risk of FFS being preauthorized and then subsequently denied reimbursement due to the lack of benefit coverage. This is also important for protecting a patient from significant financial liability if coverage were to be denied.

Some insurance carriers may balk at the request for a single case agreement by in-network surgeons given the already established participation contract but FFS does not have a defined set of CPT codes and many CPT codes used are unlisted CPT codes, which do not have agreed on reimbursements in most standard participation agreements. As such, it is reasonable for in-network surgeons to obtain single case agreements to define coverage and reimbursement for transgender patients undergoing FFS.

CURRENT PROCEDURAL TERMINOLOGY CODING FOR FACIAL FEMINIZATION SURGERY

CPT coding for FFS is difficult and controversial. There is not a defined set of CPT codes that accurately describe or represent feminizing procedures or the skill set and training to safely complete FFS. This lack of standard is emphasized in the insurance realm because varying insurance carriers and even policies within the same insurance carrier network allow or disallow certain CPT coding for FFS.[10–12,15,16] In addition, as described above, many facial feminization surgeons and insurance carriers use unlisted CPT codes in combination with listed CPT codes. Please note that despite a surgeon using a certain set or group of CPT codes for FFS, each insurance contract may have varying policies for what codes can be used. This creates an issue of what codes to submit for approval, associated billed charges, reimbursement, and creating an overall consistent billing method for the practice and patient. It is recommended that any surgeon obtaining approval for FFS carefully review the insurance's utilization management guidelines on gender-affirming services before submitting for preauthorization and predetermination. A surgeon may use certain CPT codes for one insurance carrier and a different set of CPT codes for another carrier based on the separate insurance carrier's policies. The lack of coding standard also reiterates the importance for single case agreements before rendering facial feminization surgical services.

AMENDMENTS/CARVE OUTS TO PARTICIPATION AGREEMENTS

For surgeons and practices that have higher surgical volume for facial gender-affirming services, obtaining an amendment or carve out agreement with insurers for these procedures is reasonable. Coordinating and obtaining multiple single case agreements can be time consuming and cumbersome for both insurance practice representatives and administrative staffing. A carve out agreement is a contract between an insurance carrier and the practice defining what diagnosis codes and CPT codes will be used for FFS and the agreed on reimbursement for those codes. Having a carve out will reduce the administrative workload and provide some legal and financial recourse should reimbursement not occur. However, surgeons will likely need to demonstrate a certain amount of surgical volume with an insurance carrier before taking this next step. Insurers may also be hesitant to complete this amendment given the variation in coverage policies for gender-affirming surgeries and the lack of standard for CPT coding. Amendments similar to global participation agreements are subject to revision, and termination under defined terms and time frames.

INSURANCE CLAIM SUBMISSION AND ADJUDICATION

Insurance claim submission, adjudication, and finally remittance remain challenging for many gender-affirming surgeons. Submission of claims can be completed electronically, via mail, or manually entered by insurance representatives. Some practices also use third party billing administrators to aid with this component of their practice. The method of claim entry depends on each practice's preference and resources available. Most carriers with paper-based claim submissions require the standard CMS-1500 billing form. The claim submitted however, regardless of method, should include all of the necessary documentation to support the claim submission. Recommended documents to include are (1) preauthorization documentation including all authorized CPT codes, (2) predetermination documentation or evidence of benefit coverage, (3) signed/executed single case agreement, (4) completed CMS-1500 form with listed CPT codes and associated billed charges, and (5) operative report. Even when providing the supporting documentation, there is high likelihood that adjudication and remittance will be error prone. The application of multiprocedure discounts or the exclusion of codes based on insurers gender-affirming treatment policies can alter expected reimbursement. Having a dedicated billing team to follow-up on these claims or file the necessary appeals is often required. Single case agreements help provide documentation for agreed on reimbursement associated with FFS and are highly recommended.

SUMMARY

Insurance coverage for facial gender-affirming surgeries is complex. Access to insurance coverage for these services needs continued expansion, although the decision for surgeons to work with insurers remains an individually based decision.

CLINICS CARE POINTS

- Insurance approval for gender-affirming care requires persistence and a well coordinated pre-certification team
- Obtaining written documentation of benefit coverage for gender affirming surgery is a requirement prior to completing facial feminization surgery
- Close monitoring and follow-up on insurance claim adjudication should occur to avoid error prone reimbursement processing

DISCLOSURES

The author does not have any financial disclosures or conflicts of interest related to the presented publication.

REFERENCES

1. Ngaage LM, McGlone KL, Xue S, et al. Gender surgery beyond chest and genitals: current insurance landscape. Aesthetic Surg J 2020;40:NP202–10.
2. Hu AC, Dang BC, Bertrand AA, et al. Insurance barriers and appeals for facial feminization surgery: a cost-analysis. J Am Coll Surg 2020;231:S228.
3. Ngaage LM, Knighton BJ, McGlone KL, et al. Health insurance coverage of gender-affirming top surgery in the United States. Plast Reconstr Surg 2019;144:824–33.
4. Gorbea E, Gidumal S, Kozato A, et al. Insurance coverage of facial gender affirmation surgery: a review of medicaid and commercial insurance. Otolaryngol Head Neck Surg 2021;165:791–7.
5. Gadkaree SK, DeVore EK, Richburg K, et al. National variation of insurance coverage for gender-affirming facial feminization surgery. Facial Plastic Surgery & Aesthetic Medicine 2021;23:270–7.
6. Cohen WA, Sangalang AM, Dalena MM, et al. Navigating insurance policies in the united states for gender-affirming surgery. Plast Reconstr Surg Glob Open 2019;7:e2564.
7. Hu AC, Dang BN, Bertrand AA, et al. Facial feminization surgery under insurance: the university of California Los angeles experience. Plast Reconstr Surg Glob Open 2021;9:e3572.
8. Das RK, Dusetzina SB. Gender-affirming hormone therapy spending and use in the USA, 2013–2019. J Gen Intern Med 2022. https://doi.org/10.1007/s11606-022-07693-0.
9. Coleman E, Radix AE, Bouman WP, et al. Standards of care for the health of transgender and gender diverse people, version 8. International Journal of Transgender Health 2022;23:S1–259.
10. Gender Affirming Surgery - Medical Clinical Policy Bulletins | Aetna n.d. Available at: http://www.aetna.com/cpb/medical/data/600_699/0615.html. (Accessed October 12, 2022).
11. CIGNA. Gender Dysphoria Treatment 2022. Available at: https://static.cigna.com/assets/chcp/pdf/coveragePolicies/medical/mm_0266_coverageposition criteria_gender_reassignment_surgery.pdf. Accessed October 12, 2022.
12. UHC. United Healthcare Gender Dysphoria Treatment 2022. Available at: https://www.uhcprovider.com/content/dam/provider/docs/public/policies/medicaid-comm-plan/gender-dysphoria-treatment-cs.pdf. Accessed October 12, 2022.
13. Preauthorization - Glossary. HealthCareGov n.d. Available at: https://www.healthcare.gov/glossary/preauthorization. Accessed October 12, 2022.
14. Referral, predetermination, authorization, pre-certification: What's the difference? n.d. Available at: https://www.mgma.com/resources/operations-management/guide-to-closing-a-private-equity-transaction-pre. Accessed October 12, 2022.
15. CareFirst BCBS. 7.01.123 Gender Affirmation Services. Medical Policy Reference Manual 2020. Available at: https://secure.compliance360.com/Common/ViewUploadedFile.aspx?PD=PbRt%2bA78MS7PVEIb0BPUrxmvBFa1SPU4ltdHJ34zAdg6PoPqxxQdqmbzK%2bno1gyiUBj7xXNByyFd2L5NKfHmu4ic26KI9SOqLJzWjdgopqv5ebZzTiiULLiXhf7cM%2bCmfljjQwYZWS8Ouu687kgIe27UkRiMu0Oavq1n4RFt6gMLBd1hMoRyGFCxOS1BqSC0OWoRslLQs4eQu8D1xDB2geWlAHv06EJaxXX2Yfu9txaTJkUjaMP1BeSSL%2fz5rMBKH8eXloCaKVFX4IX1vbgKAi98onnTCh3c. Accessed October 26, 2022.
16. Anthem BCBS. UM Clincal Guideline: CG-SURG-27 Gender Affirming Surgery n.d. Available at: https://www.anthem.com/dam/medpolicies/abc/active/guidelines/gl_pw_a051166.html. Accessed October 26, 2022.

Gender-Affirmation Hair Transplantation Techniques

Anthony Bared, MD*, Jeffrey S. Epstein, MD

KEYWORDS

• Hair restoration • Hairline • Eyebrow • Follicular unit extraction

INTRODUCTION

Hair restoration can play an important role for transgender patients seeking gender-affirmation procedures. In our clinic, we have seen an increase in transgender patients seeking hair restoration. The most common hair restoration procedures performed in our clinic for the transgender patient are hairline lowering procedures, facial hair restoration procedures including eyebrow and beard transplantation, and body hair transplantation. Hair restoration can be an important component for the male-to-female (MTF) transgender patient as part of the gender transformation as the rounding of a hairline, for instance, can help to provide for a more feminine appearance as does creating an arched shape to the eyebrows. For the female-to-male (FTM) patient, beard and chest hair transplantation helps to create a more masculine facial and body appearance. In this article, we present our experience in hair restoration for the transgender patient. We review the best candidates for hair restoration as it relates to the transgender patient, the techniques which provide for the most natural results, and the postoperative course from hair transplantation.

PREOPERATIVE PLANNING
Consultation

The consultation for hair restoration serves to attain a medical and hair loss history to ascertain the patient's goals for a procedure, provide for a proper examination of the scalp donor hair and recipient area, and establish mutual goals for the procedure. A hair loss-specific questionnaire is completed by the patient before the consultation, and this is reviewed with the patient at the time of consultation. Hair loss history needs to be obtained if there is androgenic hair loss evident in the patient as well as a family history of hair loss. In the MTF patient taking hormonal therapy or having undergone gender reassignment, there is no further risk of potential future male pattern hair loss. An examination of the scalp, paying close attention to the quality of the donor hair, needs to be performed. The donor hair needs to be examined for its quality and density so as to estimate the number of grafts that may be obtained in a procedure as well as over the course of the patient's lifetime. When reviewing the patient's goals for the procedure whether hairline lowering or facial hair restoration, it is often helpful that the patient brings model photos of their "ideal" outcome to review at the time of the consultation. We do not perform computerized imaging for hair restoration as we find that this gives unrealistic expectations from surgery, but instead mark out photos of the patient, drawing in for them the potential position of their hairline or beard shape. As in any area of esthetic surgery, proper expectations need to be established and understood, whether it is the degree of hairline lowering possible through a single procedure, or the amount of density attainable in either hairline lowering or facial hair transplantation. Risks of the procedure are reviewed with the patient. Last, of course, patients need to be in generally good medical health to undergo a procedure.

Private Practice, Facial Plastic Surgery and Hair Restoration, 6280 Sunset Drive, Suite 504, Miami, FL 33143, USA
* Corresponding author.
E-mail address: abared@dranthonybared.com

Facial Plast Surg Clin N Am 31 (2023) 375–380
https://doi.org/10.1016/j.fsc.2023.04.003

Hairline Design

Although hairline designs vary tremendously, the important goal is that of achieving a natural-appearing female hairline. When designing a hairline for the transgender patient, multiple factors need to be considered. The position of the existing hairline, the presence of androgenic alopecia, family history of hair loss, use of hormonal therapy such as finasteride or estrogens, and the density and quality of the donor hair are all factors to keep in mind.[1] In general, feminizing a hairline entails the lowering of the hairline and the blunting of the temporal region.[2] A soft, "heart-shaped" hairline design with rounded recession in the frontal–temporal region (Fig. 1) is often used to feminize the hairline and achieve a natural appearance to the hairline.[3] To aid in the creation of a natural hairline appearance, oftentimes a subtle widow's peak is created slightly off center. Rounding of the hairline is then performed posteriorly and laterally along the frontal–temporal region, connecting to the temporal points. This design helps to soften the hairline, blunt the temporal area, and feminize the hairline. On the day of the procedure, the patient is met in the preoperative suite where her hairline is marked out using a washable surgical marking pen. The patients are then shown the hairline design in front of a mirror. Preoperative photos are taken before and after the markings.

Beard Design

Goals in beard design are often established by the patient. Many patients typically present with a rather specific understanding of how they want their facial hair to appear. The design and density of the beard may be limited by the quality of the donor hair. The transplantation of full beards requires a large amount of grafts and patients are always made aware of the possibility of undergoing secondary procedures after around 1 year if further density is desired. It is our experience that the scalp hair transplants to the face have a very high regrowth percentage and if properly performed patients can achieve a very natural outcome. Depending on the exact design and density, graft counts can range from 600 to 1000 grafts per cheek/sideburn area and 400 to 800 grafts to the mustache and goatee. Using the patient's guidelines, the areas to be transplanted are marked out using a surgical marking pen with the patient in a seated position. The markings are checked for symmetry between the two sides. Measurements are used to help ensure symmetry. The patient is shown the markings in a mirror. If then needed, alterations are made according to patient desires (Fig. 2).

Eyebrow Design

When approaching eyebrow restoration for the transgender patient, it is important to appreciate the shape of the more masculine eyebrow versus that of a more feminine eyebrow appearance. The masculine eyebrow shape is generally less arched but rather comes to a lateral widening at the peak of the brow, whereas the feminine eyebrow shape is more rounded and arched (Fig. 3A, B). The goal in eyebrow restoration for the transgender patient wishing to create a more feminine appearance is to create an arched-shaped appearance to the eyebrows, whereas in all patients, the goals are to provide the desired shape, density, natural direction, and angle of growth of eyebrow hair. Patients are encouraged to bring in photos of their "ideal" or model eyebrows. On the day of the procedure, the patient is first seen in the preoperative suite where photos are taken. Preoperative photography is very important in eyebrow transplantation as it truly helps to provide for another means of visualizing

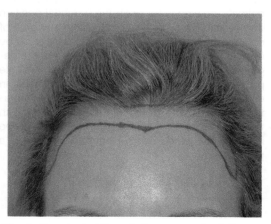

Fig. 1. Female hairline design generally follows a "heart-shaped" design with slight rounding in the frontal–temporal region.

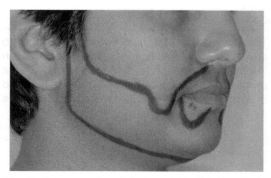

Fig. 2. An example of a beard design as drawn preoperatively.

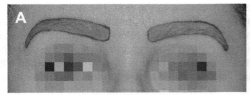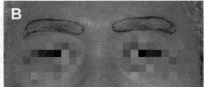

Fig. 3. (*A*) Female eyebrow design. (*B*) Male eyebrow design with a lateral widening and a non-arched design.

the planned eyebrow shape before the procedure. Photos are taken of the patient both with eyes open and closed. It is often found that eyebrow elevation is asymmetric as there tends to be an asymmetric elevation of the eyebrows by the facial musculature and sometimes that associated with asymmetry of the eyelids. These asymmetries are noted and also made known to the patient. Preliminary drawings are made by the patient if desired with an eyeliner pencil. Once preliminary drawings are made by the patient, the surgeon then fine tunes the shape. Measurements are taken along the length and in various places along the width of the eyebrows to ensure as much symmetry as possible. The midline is marked and measurements of the midline are also taken. The final shape is then shown to the patient, and photos of this shape are taken in a similar fashion to the premarking photos.

SURGICAL PROCEDURE
Donor Hair Harvest

In the majority of all hair transplants we perform, the donor hairs are harvested by the follicular unit extraction (FUE) technique, which avoids altogether a linear donor site incision and thus patients are able to cut the hair typically as short as desired.[4] However, we still occasionally perform, particularly in females including MTF transgender hair transplants, use the "strip" method for harvesting the donor hairs. The "strip" method avoids the need for significant shaving of the back and sometimes sides of the head that is typically needed for large FUE procedures. However, we also use a no-shave or long-hair FUE technique, where the donor hair is extracted via the FUE method, whereas the surrounding hairs in the donor area are maintained long and not needed to be entirely trimmed. This is a more tedious procedure but allows for FUE extraction, avoiding a linear scar, and allows for the patient to maintain their hair long.

Hairline

The position and shape of the hairline is, at first, drawn for the patient using a removable ink marking pen. The patient is shown the hairline design in front of a mirror. Once the position and shape of the hairline is determined, photos are taken of the design and the markings are reinforced with a permanent ink marker so as not to be lost during the procedure. Most patients are then given oral anxiolytic medication.

The goal of hairline lowering is to create the most natural-appearing results by replicating the direction and angle of the existing hairline. The smallest possible incisions are made allowing for the placement of the hair grafts. The one, two, and three hair grafts are tested to ensure size compatibility with the recipient sites. Acute angulation of the grafts is important particularly in the first few rows of the hairline. Depending on the characteristics of the hair—thickness and curl—typically the first two to three rows are composed of single hair grafts placed in an irregular pattern, followed by the placement of two- to three-hair grafts. The central portion of the hairline is the area that tends to be most dense, so it is important that the central aspect is adequately filled to allow for the creation of the most density in this region. As mentioned, the direction of hair growth follows the existing hairline, but most commonly, hairs are placed with an acute forward direction on the central region and then tapered down/inferiorly along the temples (**Fig. 4**). The grafts are then placed in the incisions with implanter devices that minimize trauma to the grafts and can expedite the planting process.

Patients are explained to expect swelling along the forehead and eyes for 1 to 2 days after the

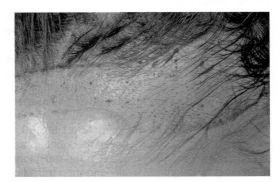

Fig. 4. Intraoperative photo of the direction and angulation of the female hairline graft placement.

procedure. They are seen in the office on postoperative day number one for a hair wash and are explained how to wash the hair and care for the grafts. Light washings are performed without allowing the shower water to directly hit the grafts for the first 6 days after surgery followed by normal showers after that point. The crusts are to be gently removed after 6 days.

Beard

Currently, in our practice, nearly all patients seeking facial hair restoration elect to have the grafts obtained via the FUE technique. In these cases, the donor area is shaved (unless a no-shave approach is used) and patients are placed in a supine position. The smallest possible drill size avoiding graft transection is used for the extractions. The donor area consists of the occiput only in smaller cases and extends into the parietal scalp for larger cases. Once the extractions have been completed from the occipital area, the patient is then turned to lie in the supine position.

Local anesthesia is then applied to the face starting in each sideburn and cheek area. The perioral region is not anesthetized at this point but rather the area around the mouth is typically worked on after the patient has eaten lunch. The recipient sites in the sideburn and cheek area are made first. The smallest possible recipient sites are made using 0.5, 0.6, and sometimes 0.7 mm slits. In the periphery of the sideburns, one-hair grafts are used, whereas two-hair grafts can be placed in the central aspect of the sideburn to allow for more density. It is imperative to make the incisions at an ultra-acute angle to the skin. The direction of the growth is generally downward, but more centrally closer to the mouth/goatee region can be somewhat anterior. In the cheek area, mostly one- and two-hair grafts are used; however, in the occasional patient with fine donor hair, some three-hair grafts can be used to allow for the achievement of greater density. As soon as recipient site formation is done, the grafts can then be placed one at a time, according to the vision of the surgeon.

After the patient is given lunch, the area around the mouth is then anesthetized. Infraorbital and mental nerve blocks are used to provide initial anesthesia. The goatee and mustache area anesthesia is then reinforced with field subdermal local anesthesia complemented by epinephrine 1:50,000 to minimize bleeding. Incisions in the goatee and mustache area are then made. On the mustache, hairs will grow slightly laterally and then transition downward along the goatee. Once again, it is very important to make these at an acute an angle as

possible to the skin. The grafts in the mustache region have the tendency to grow perpendicular; thus, patients need to be made aware of the difficulty in creating density along the entire mustache, particularly centrally within the "cupid's bow." The creation of density in this area is difficult owing to the topography created by the upper lip's "cupid's bow" area. The transition from the mustache to the goatee is an important area for the creation of density, which is usually created by the maximal dense packing of two hair grafts.

Graft placement continues, and toward the conclusion of the case, the patient is given a mirror before all grafts are placed. Given that the immediate results closely replicate the final results, it is helpful for the patient to view the beard in order to assess the design and density of the grafts. This allows for feedback, fine-tuning, and alteration before the conclusion of the case (**Fig. 5**).

Patients are to keep the face dry for the first 5 days after the procedure. This allows for the grafts to set properly, helping assure the maintenance of proper angulation. Topical antibiotic ointment is applied to the donor area whether a strip or FUE technique was used. Patients are then to wet the face after 5 days with soap and water, starting to remove the dried blood and crusts. Shaving is permitted after 10 days.

Eyebrow

The donor area is anesthetized with local anesthesia composed of lidocaine 2%/1:100,000 epinephrine. These grafts can be obtained by the strip or FUE technique. Given the relatively small number of grafts needed for eyebrow transplantation, the no-shave FUE technique can easily be used for these patients electing to not have the strip method while allowing the surrounding hair to be maintained long.

Once the donor hairs have been harvested, the patient is then placed in a seated, reclined position

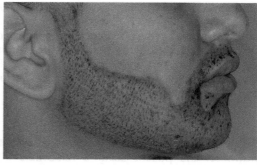

Fig. 5. Immediate postoperative photo of patient in **Fig. 2** showing beard hair graft placement.

for incision site formation. The eyebrow area is anesthetized with local anesthesia containing epinephrine for hemostasis. The recipient sites are made using the smallest blade size for the graft—typically 0.5 or 0.6 mm. The initial recipient sites are made along the periphery along the pre-marked borders of the eyebrows. It is important to start with these peripheral marking incisions as the preoperative markings can soon be lost with the subsequent bleeding and wiping. Incisions are made at an acute angle as possible to the skin (Fig. 6). Within the medial-most aspect of the eyebrow inferiorly, the hairs usually grow in a superior and slightly lateral direction. As one moves more superior within the head of the eyebrow, the direction changes to a more lateral and then inferior direction. As one then moves more laterally into the body (midportion), the hairs grow in an inferior-lateral direction along the superior border and in a superior-lateral direction along the inferior border. Within this body, which constitutes the majority of the eyebrow, this crossed-hatch pattern achieves the greatest amount of density. Then, the lateral-most one-quarter or so of the eyebrow, called the tail, has typically horizontally oriented recipient sites.

Once all incision sites are made, the grafts are then inserted. A typical procedure can range from 150 to as many as 400 grafts per eyebrow. The grafts are placed so that the direction of the hair growth, that is, the curl of the hair, is placed to complement the goal of having the hairs grow in as an acute angle as possible with the skin. In most cases, as many two-hair grafts as possible are placed within the eyebrows, primarily the central portion but also in parts of the head. Two-hair grafts are not used if the hairs within a graft are divergent in their growth. The utilization of as many two-hair grafts as possible creates the most amount of density within the eyebrows. Mostly one-hair grafts are used along the borders, periphery, and tail region.

After all the grafts are placed, the patient is asked to sit up and the eyebrows are inspected. Additional grafts are then placed if small adjustments are deemed appropriate. The patient is then shown the eyebrows in a mirror for feedback as well (Fig. 7).

Patients are instructed to maintain the eyebrow area dry for 5 days. The scalp hair may be washed the first postoperative day. Antibiotic ointment is applied to the donor area twice daily for 1 week. Patients are allowed to use makeup in the eyebrow area after all the crusts have fallen out at typically 5 to 7 days.

Chest and Other Pubic Region

There are a variety of indications for performing these body hair procedures. Chest hair procedures can both serve to create a more masculine appearance, but also to help conceal mastectomy scars in MTF patients. Pubic hair transplants are primarily indicated in patients who have undergone gender reassignment, where the normal escutcheon can similarly help conceal any scarring (Fig. 8).

For the chest, the procedures of 1800 to as many as 3000 grafts are indicated due to the relatively large area that needs to be covered. These potential areas, depending on patient goals, can include the upper and central chest, ranging laterally and inferiorly (particularly to conceal mastectomy scars), and even continue caudally in a vertical direction into the abdomen and even upper pubic region. The keys to achieving a natural result, besides careful acute angulation of the recipient sites, are to have a crossed-hatch pattern of hair growth toward the midline, that is, sternum.

A crossed-hatch pattern centrally—to achieve the greatest appearance of density—is also indicated when performing pubic hair transplants.

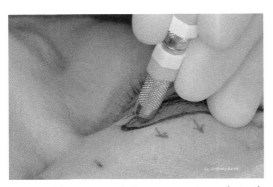

Fig. 6. Incisions are made in a very acute angle to the skin with 0.5 to 0.6 mm blades.

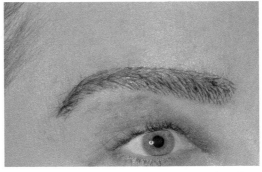

Fig. 7. Immediate postoperative results of eyebrow transplantation.

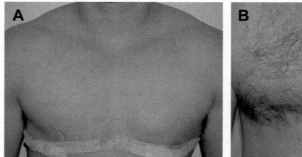
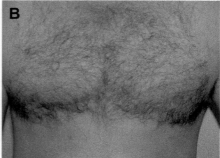

Fig. 8. (*A, B*) Before and after 2000 grafts to chest—FTM patient—to create a more masculine appearance and conceal mastectomy scars.

Typical procedures range from 400 to 900 grafts, depending on the patient's goals in terms of density and area covered.

SUMMARY

Hairline patterns and facial hair distribution can be gender-identifying traits. Females tend to have a lower and more rounded hairline than men as well have more arched brows, whereas males, of course, have a prevalence of facial hair. Hair transplantation can play a complementary role for the transgender patient undergoing gender transformation. In our clinic, the most common hair transplantations seen in the transgender patient are hairline lowering, beard transplantation, and eyebrow transplantation. Although challenging from an artistic and

technical perspective, these procedures have a very high satisfaction rate for the patients.

REFERENCES

1. Rogers N. Imposters of Androgenic Alopecia. Facial Plast Surg Clin N Am 2013;21:325–34.
2. Rassman WR, et al. Phenotype of Normal Hairline Maturation. Facial Plast Surg Clin N Am 2013;21:317–24.
3. Nausbaum BP, Fuentefria S. Naturally occurring female hairline patterns. Dermatol Surg 2009;35:907–13.
4. Rassman WR, Berstein RM, McClellan R, et al. Follicular Unit Extraction: minimally invasive surgery for hair transplantation. Dermatol Surg 2002;28:720–8.

Gender-Affirming Surgery of the Mandible
Lower Jaw Feminization and Masculinization

Benjamin B. Massenburg, MD[a,b], Russell E. Ettinger, MD[a,b], Shane D. Morrison, MD, MS[a,b,*]

KEYWORDS

- Gender affirming • Mandible contouring • Genioplasty • Lower jaw augmentation • Chin implants
- Osteotomies • Craniofacial surgery

KEY POINTS

- Lower jaw feminization typically consists of bony reduction and contouring of the mandibular angle and body along with genioplasty for shortening, narrowing, and possible advancement or lengthening depending on a patient's facial morphology.
- Lower jaw masculinization consists of augmentation with alloplastic implants, bone grafts, or fat grafting over the mandibular angle and body, and chin augmentation with alloplastic implants, genioplasty, or fat grafting.
- Complications are uncommon but can be significant if there is a mandible fracture, nerve injury, implant infection, or other surgical site infection.
- Standardized guidelines are needed for safe and effective surgical pathways for facial gender-affirming surgery.

 Video content accompanies this article at http://www.facialplastic.theclinics.com.

INTRODUCTION

For patients with gender dysphoria, gender-affirming surgery of the face has continued to advance over the last 35 years, since Dr Douglas Ousterhout published his seminal article in 1987.[1] The literature shows that facial feminization surgery is much more common than facial masculinization surgery, likely due to the powerful masculinizing effects of testosterone. Of the aspects of facial feminization surgery, lower jaw contouring tends to be the least commonly performed surgery, when compared to the forehead and midface. This article will review the literature on gender-affirming surgery of the lower jaw, both facial feminization and facial masculinization, and both bony contouring and soft tissue adjunctive procedures.

There are several key differences in the bony and soft tissue architecture of the feminine and masculine face, as highlighted in **Table 1**. Focusing on the lower jaw, there is increased mandibular body height, increased gonial splay, and a gonial angle typically less than 125° in the masculine mandible (**Figs. 1–4**). The chin is typically larger, wider, and squarer in the masculine mandible (see **Figs. 1** and **4**; **Fig. 5**). All of these differences can be addressed with gender-affirming craniofacial surgery of the mandible.

a Division of Plastic Surgery, Department of Surgery, University of Washington; b Division of Craniofacial and Plastic Surgery, Department of Surgery, Seattle Children's Hospital
* Corresponding author. Division of Plastic and Reconstructive Surgery, Department of Surgery, Harborview Medical Center, 325 9th Avenue, Mailstop #359796, Seattle, WA 98104.
E-mail address: shanedm@uw.edu

Facial Plast Surg Clin N Am 31 (2023) 381–392
https://doi.org/10.1016/j.fsc.2023.04.001
1064-7406/23/© 2023 Elsevier Inc. All rights reserved.

Table 1
Phenotypic differences between the feminine and masculine face

Phenotypes	Feminine	Masculine
Face Shape[40]	Rounded and soft appearing, heart or inverted triangle shape	Angulated and square, with a pronounced jaw and chin
Hairline[41]	Lower, gentle curve, convex	Higher, M-shaped with temporal hairline recession
Frontal Bossing[1]	Smooth continuously round contour of frontal bone	Pronounced bony supraorbital ridge
Eyebrows[42]	Laterally peaked, above the superior orbital rim	Straight, on the superior orbital rim
Naso-Frontal Angle[43]	Obtuse	Acute
Nose[43]	Thin-based and concave, Supratip break, narrower dorsal esthetic lines	Wide and straight or convex, minimal Supratip break, convex dorsal esthetic lines
Lips[12]	Fuller vermilion, shorter cutaneous height, with more incisal show	Thin vermilion and elongated cutaneous upper lip, with less incisal show
Occlusal Plane[13]	More neutral occlusal plane	Flatter occlusal plane
Mandible[44]	Reduced mandibular body height	Increased mandibular body height, increased gonial splay
Gonial Angle[45]	Greater than 125°	<125°
Chin[45]	Small, pointed, or rounded, 20% shorter than in males[46]	Large, wide, square
Masseter[47,48]	Smaller muscle bulk	Bulky muscle
Thyroid Cartilage[49,50]	120° angle of cartilage	90° angle of cartilage

PREOPERATIVE ASSESSMENT

As transgender health and surgery advances toward equity, The World Professional Association for Transgender Health (WPATH) has published updates to their Standards of Care (SOC) since 1979,[2] with the goal of providing clinical guidance for safe and effective medical and surgical pathways for gender diverse people. Version 7 of the SOC, published in 2012, did not explicitly define the medical necessity of facial gender-affirmation surgery.[3,4] However, there have been several studies that show facial feminization can improve the feminine perception of the face,[5,6] improve quality of life,[7] and reduce misgendering.[8] Harmonizing a patient's facial form with their gender identity can also limit the patient's risk for targeting and interpersonal violence based on facial anatomic incongruence with an individual's gender identity.

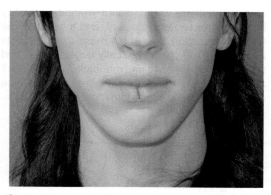

Fig. 1. Preoperative frontal view of a patient planning on undergoing lower jaw facial feminization surgery.

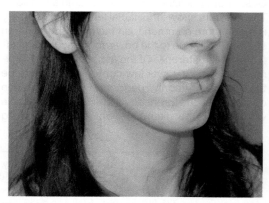

Fig. 2. Preoperative three-quarter view of a patient planning on undergoing lower jaw facial feminization surgery.

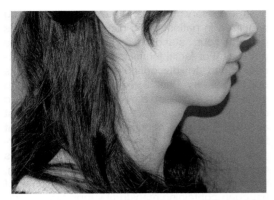

Fig. 3. Preoperative right facial view of a patient planning on undergoing lower jaw facial feminization surgery.

Thus, there have been several international groups that have studied and advocated for the medical necessity of facial gender-affirming surgery,[3,9] which has since been included as medically indicated in the WPATH SOC Version 8.[10]

Preoperatively, patients will meet with their mental health provider and primary care provider before a surgical evaluation. The mental health provider will be able to thoroughly evaluate the patient's gender dysphoria and treat or support any comorbid mental health issue. Evaluation by their primary care provider will optimize any underlying medical conditions which could negatively impact the surgical outcomes. Generally, we prefer patients to have made a medical transition and have completed 1 year of hormone therapy, if they can safely do so and hormones are part of their gender identity. This allows for maximal end-organ effects of testosterone or estrogen to modify the skin and soft tissues so that the remaining dysphoric facial features that cannot be improved with hormone therapy can be identified and addressed directly with surgical intervention.[11]

A thorough preoperative dental and orthodontic evaluation should be performed in all cases with identification of baseline dentofacial disharmony, malocclusion, and the dental show being noted as these can have a dramatic effect on the perception of gender.[12,13] Treatment of dental caries or gingival disease preoperatively is essential to reduce the risk of infection.[14] If planning for orthognathic surgery, the patient must also be evaluated for the presence of third molars which may impact the osteotomy site.[15] Ideally, all patients under consideration for osseous facial gender-affirming surgery procedures should have attained skeletal maturity to assure the longevity of their final post-operative results.

Following these multidisciplinary consultations, the surgical team should additionally evaluate the medical, medication, dental, gender, and mental health history of the patient and also evaluate their face as a whole to determine the feminine and masculine characteristics, while listening to the patient's main areas of concern. Focusing on the lower third of the face, it is important to assess the occlusion, incisal show, bony prominence of the mandible including gonial splay, mandibular body prominence, chin vertical height, and sagittal projection for prognathism or retrognathism. Following skeletal assessment, it is also essential to examine the soft tissue envelope, mimetic muscle thickness, masseter muscle bulk at rest and with masticatory effort, prominent submandibular glands, evidence of prior soft tissue augmentation (fillers) or scarring, and the degree of generalized facial aging as evidence by soft tissue ptosis, perioral rhytids, nasojugal grooving, jowling as well as assessing the overall skin texture and

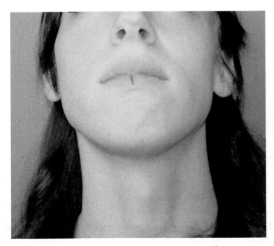

Fig. 4. Preoperative worm's eye view of a patient planning on undergoing lower jaw facial feminization surgery.

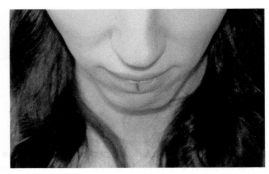

Fig. 5. Preoperative bird's eye view of a patient planning on undergoing lower jaw facial feminization surgery.

quality as these features will inform the need for either skeletal reduction or augmentation to assure optimal surgical results.

Standard preoperative facial photographs should be taken as these are often required when seeking insurance approvals for gender-affirming facial surgery. Advanced imaging modalities, specifically computed tomographic (CT) imaging of the head, face, and neck, can assist with planning of any osteotomies, bony contouring, bony augmentation, and identification of critical anatomic landmarks and facilitate surgical case execution. If pursuing preoperative virtual surgical planning, computer-aided design, or computer-aided manufacturing of cutting guides, splints, or osteosynthesis materials, CT imaging is essential (**Fig. 6**).[16] Our experience is in alignment with the existing research that has shown that the use of cutting guides for mandibular contouring and genioplasty decreases operative times and allows extremely precise and predictable results.[17]

Once the decision has been made to pursue surgery, all risks should be disclosed to the patient. These include risks of wound dehiscence, infection, osteomyelitis, dental injury, sensory nerve neuropraxias, or permanent paresthesia. Patients with active nicotine use are not candidates for facial gender-confirming procedures as the risk of complications is not trivial due to the vasoconstrictive effects and heat generated with smoking or vape delivery methods. Urine cotinine screening is utilized in patients with nicotine use history as part of our standard presurgical clearance pathway. For facial feminization surgery, it is recommended to discontinue estrogen 3 weeks before surgery until 3 weeks after surgery to decrease the risk of a venous thromboembolic event, yet definitive data on this are not robust and some centers continue estrogen throughout facial feminization. For facial masculinization surgery, testosterone can be continued but does carry an anecdotal increased risk of bleeding, but individuals are also assessed for the use of estrogen-containing menstrual suppression medications and a shared decision-making process is used to determine if they will be stopped or continued.

FACIAL FEMINIZATION

Preoperative planning should be performed weeks before the surgical date, to ensure adequate fabrication and transit time for any cutting guides or patient-specific fixation materials (see **Fig. 6**). Modification of the mandible and lower third of the face for facial feminization can be combined with other midfacial, upper facial, and nasal procedures, so the method of airway securement can vary, but we prefer an orotracheal intubation with the endotracheal (ET) tube secured to a maxillary first molar with a 26 gauge circumdental wire.

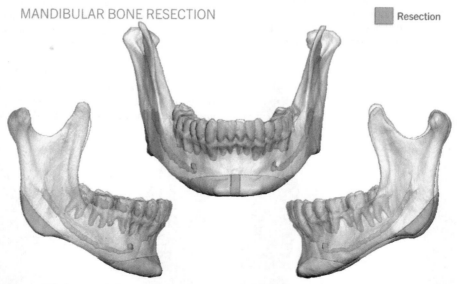

MANDIBULAR BONE RESECTION   Resection

Fig. 6. Computer-aided surgical planning with the use of CT images for mandibular angle ostectomy and narrowing genioplasty allows for visualization of the inferior alveolar nerve along its entire course. In this patient, we planned bony reduction of the transverse and vertical jaw dimensions and softening of the gonial angles with an ostectomy of the buccal and lingual cortices of the mandibular angle, along with a narrowing and advancing genioplasty.

Before definitively securing the ET tube, the patient's neck is fully extended and flexed with the anesthesia team ensuring that ventilation is maintained throughout all positions, and once confirmed, the tube is fully secured with the surgical wire. A throat pack is placed in the pharynx, and the teeth are cleansed and brushed with chlorhexidine mouthwash. Antibiotics with oral flora coverage (ampicillin/sulbactam) are given preoperatively and re-dosed as indicated for time. The patient's face, head, and neck are typically prepped circumferentially with antibiotic irrigation given the need for a full head, hairline, face, and neck exposure for concurrent multilevel facial gender-affirming surgery procedures.

Key intraoral anatomic landmarks including the location of Stenson's ducts as well as the approximate location of the mental nerve should be noted and marked before designing incisions. The incision should be marked wide on the gingival mucosa to ensure that there is an adequate cuff of mucosa for closure. The length and position of the incisions are predicated on what regions of the mandible are going to be accessed to perform osteotomies or bony contouring. Some prefer to completely expose the mandible from angle to angle,[18] while others prefer a three-incision approach at the symphysis and bilateral body/angle region that are tunneled to connect subperiosteally, leaving a cuff of mucosa overlying the mental nerve as a way to reduce incisional burden.[19] Once incisions have been planned and marked, local anesthetic with epinephrine is given along the course of the planned incision for analgesic and vasoconstrictive effects.

Mandibular Angle and Body Contouring

After incision through the mucosa, the dissection is continued directly onto the buccal cortex of the mandible using monopolar electrocautery. Once down to the bone, a periosteal incision is carried out with electrocautery and subperiosteal dissection is used to expose the mandibular angle if gonial angle osteotomies or contouring is to be performed. Mesial extension of this incision toward the mental nerve can be completed to allow for exposure of the mandibular body if buccal cortex or inferior border contouring is required. When using cutting guides, it may be necessary to dissect a larger area to allow for the added bulk of a cutting guide and to allow for bone adaptation in the subperiosteal space (Fig. 7).

Once adequate exposure has been obtained, the bony contouring can include reduction of the transverse and/or vertical jaw dimensions and softening of the gonial angles (Fig. 8). This can

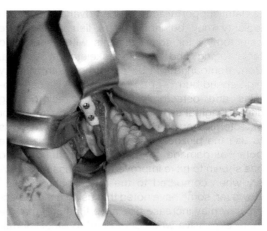

Fig. 7. Surgical approach to the right angle of the mandible through a lower gingivobuccal sulcus incision. The patient-specific cutting guide for a mandibular angle ostectomy is fixed in place before the ostectomy.

entail ostectomy of the buccal and lingual cortices of the mandibular angle in isolation to increase the gonial angle and reduce gonial splay (Video 1) versus a complete reduction of the height of the mandible from angle to angle to shorten the vertical height of the lower third of the face.[19] When planning for aggressive bony reduction, one should always consider the reciprocal destabilizing effects on the overlying soft tissue envelope. For patients with generalized facial aging and premorbid soft tissue ptosis, aggressive reductive ostectomies can result in iatrogenic worsening of facial aesthetics and yield undesirable results. Consideration for selective expansion of the

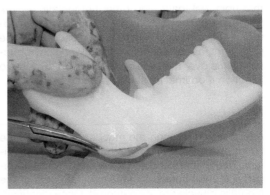

Fig. 8. Intra-operative photograph of the right mandibular angle ostectomy, as compared to a model of the patient's pre-operative mandibular morphology. Ostectomy included both buccal and lingual cortices of the mandibular angle reducing the transverse and vertical jaw dimensions and softening the gonial angles.

skeletal support via narrowing advancement genioplasty may be indicated in lieu of reductive ostectomies for some patients with generalized facial aging and baseline skeletal hypoplasia. Bony contouring can be performed with a rotary high-speed burr,[20] or a power rasp while osteotomies and ostectomies with the reciprocating saw,[21] sagittal saw, or a piezoelectric saw.[19] For ostectomies and osteotomies, our preference is to use the piezoelectric saw, as it minimizes the potential damage to adjacent structures[19] and has shown to have improved neurosensory recovery when compared to the reciprocating saw.[22] However, some have noted that using a piezoelectric saw may increase operative time and may be more expensive when compared to other modalities.[23] Preoperative CT imaging can identify the path of the inferior alveolar nerve through the mandible, which is helpful in avoiding nerve injury during bony contouring or ostectomy (see **Fig. 6**).

For a bicortical ostectomy, once the initial cortical cuts have been made, an osteotome is used to complete the osteotomy. If this posterior cut is difficult to visualize, a rigid endoscope can be utilized to facilitate visualization.[19] Due to the attachments of the medial pterygoid muscle, this fragment may migrate medially once the osteotomy is complete, and it will need to be controlled and dissected free of the medial muscular attachments.

If the patient has excessive masseteric bulk, the masseter can either be directly excised or injected with botulinum toxin. However, some reduction in muscle bulk should be expected simply due to atrophy from degloving the masseter off of the mandible.[24]

The wound is then irrigated with antibiotic irrigation and hemostasis is achieved using cautery, thrombin, gel foam, and other hemostatic agents as needed. The incision is then closed with 3-0 or 4-0 absorbable suture. The closure must be watertight, as saliva pools in the lower gingivobuccal sulcus over the incision and can predispose to infection if optimal closure is not achieved.

Genioplasty

After incision through the mucosa, the transverse fibers of the orbicularis oris muscle will be identified. These fibers should be elevated from the underlying submucosa until the sagittal fibers of the mentalis muscle are encountered. Once identified, the plane of dissection is brought up off the origin of the mentalis fibers' attachment to bone such that a robust cuff of mentalis muscle is preserved to allow for later resuspension of the muscle and soft tissue during closure. Failure to leave this

cuff and resuspend the muscle can lead to a tendency toward lower lip incompetence and a "witch's chin" deformity.[25] Once the mentalis cuff has been preserved, the dissection plane is taken down directly to the bone with incision directly through the symphyseal periosteum. Subperiosteal dissection is then propagated inferiorly over the inferior border of the mandible. Often, the periosteal attachments are tenacious in the symphyseal region and may require both blunt dissection with a periosteal elevator and the use of the monopolar cautery to facilitate exposure. Once the inferior border of the mandible has been identified, it can be used as a guide to propagate the dissection postero-laterally and identify the mental foramina which can be approached inferior to superior with blunt dissection to ensure adequate protection of the nerve as it exits the foramina. Once identified, additional inferior border dissection can be performed below the nerve to connect to the posterior mandibular dissection plane if needed.

Once adequate exposure has been obtained, the genioplasty proceeds with the patient-specific goals to shorten, narrow, and/or advance or lengthen the chin (**Fig. 9**). The chin can be tapered or vertically shortened using basal ostectomies to reduce the volume or height of the chin (Video 2).[19] If the chin needs to be advanced, an osteotomy at least 5 mm inferior to the mental foramen can be performed using a traditional reciprocating or oscillating saw or with the piezoelectric saw. The genioplasty can then be secured with permanent osteosynthesis material (**Fig. 10**) which can also be customized to a desired pre-surgically planned position with a patient-specific plate. If the chin needs to be advanced, shortened, and narrowed, a T-shaped osteotomy can be performed.[26]

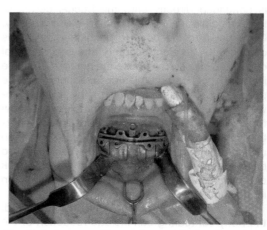

Fig. 9. Patient-specific cutting guide in place for a narrowing and advancing genioplasty.

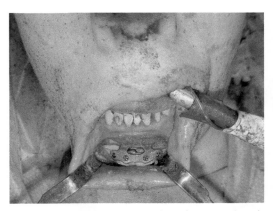

Fig. 10. Osteosynthesis material in place securing the genioplasty segments after the planned advancement and narrowing.

If the chin needs to be vertically lengthened, this can be performed with clockwise rotation of the genioplasty segment while maintaining posterior contact filling the created defect with interpositional bone grafts which can be repurposed from the gonial angle or inferior border ostectomies.[19] For augmentation, some authors have proposed using silicone chin implants, though our preference is to perform an osseous genioplasty as this provides the greatest freedom to idealize the chin position, shape, and contour and harmonize with the remainder of the facial form.[27]

Once the bony recontouring is complete, the wound is irrigated with antibiotic irrigation and hemostasis is confirmed. Before final closure, soft tissue resuspension must be performed to ensure readaptation of the overlying soft tissues to the new surgically improved mandibular contour. If a significant inferior border resection has been performed, the mylohyoid musculature resuspension can be completed using bone anchors or with drill holes along the inferior border.[19] The mentalis muscle should be reapproximated to avoid the "witch's chin" deformity.[25] The incision is then closed with 3-0 or 4-0 absorbable suture.

Preoperative and 1-month photographs of an individual who underwent mandibular angle contouring and genioplasty for mandibular facial feminization can be seen in **Figs. 11–13.**

FACIAL MASCULINIZATION

Facial masculinization is much less common than facial feminization, with sparse data in the literature and few surgeons with sizable experience.[28,29] This may be due to the profoundly masculinizing effects that exogenous testosterone can have on the facial skin texture, facial hair, and the anterior hairline which provide highly masculine facial

appearance despite a lack of skeletal masculinization.[9] Most of the literature on facial masculinization has been performed on cis-men,[30] though the techniques will be the same for trans-men.

With facial feminization being largely reductive in nature, facial masculinization is largely additive. Bone, silicone rubber, porous polyethylene, or polyetheretherketone are all materials used to augment the craniofacial skeleton in facial masculinization.[30] The approaches to the craniofacial skeleton are similar between facial feminization and facial masculinization of the lower jaw, so the airway management, surgical preparation, and draping are similar.

The incision is similarly planned wide on the gingival mucosa to ensure a large cuff of mucosa remains for closure, and local anesthetic with epinephrine is infiltrated. The mandible can either be completely degloved[18] or accessed using a three-incision approach with cuffs of mucosa surrounding the mental nerves to again limit incisional burden.[19] With alloplastic implants, meticulous watertight closures are essential to avoid implant infection placed through lower buccal sulcus approaches.

Mandibular Angle Augmentation

When dissecting the angle of the mandible, care is taken to protect the pterygomasseteric musculature, as this is the vascular supply to the mandible in this area. To maximize the bone graft survival and wound healing around implants, adequate blood supply is essential.

Implants are designed to make the gonial angle more acute and produce a squarer lower jaw. They should be tapered appropriately along the body of the mandible. Before placing the implants, the authors prefer to thoroughly irrigate the wound with antibiotic irrigation and avoid any contact between the mucosa and the implant to reduce the contamination from intraoral bacteria. The implants are secured to the mandible with monocortical screws, and the incision is closed with 3-0 or 4-0 absorbable sutures. Watertight closure remains essential as saliva will pool in the lower gingivobuccal sulcus over the incision.

Another method for mandibular angle augmentation is autologous bone grafting from the iliac crest or calvarium. Mandibular augmentation with autologous onlay grafts between the mandible and the masseter results in bone resorption,[28] so the grafts should be placed interpositionally at the angle of the mandible. The buccal cortex is split from the angle and body of the mandible while maintaining the insertions of the masseter muscle, and the remaining mandible consists of an intact

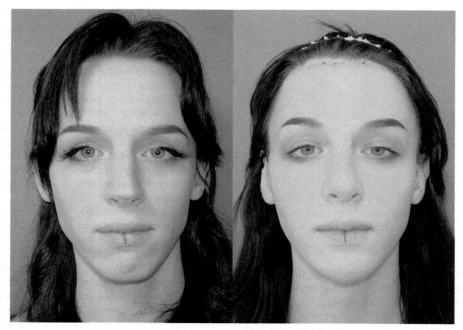

Fig. 11. Preoperative and 1-month postoperative frontal view of the same patient from **Figs. 1–5** after undergoing mandibular angle reduction and advancement and narrowing genioplasty.

alveolar arch in continuity with condyle. The authors prefer to make this split with the piezoelectric saw and complete the inferior split with an osteotome. It is important to leave the inferior pterygomandibular ligament intact to maintain stability of the mandible. The bone graft is inserted in place and secured with osteosynthesis material. Donor site morbidity as well as bony resorption should be discussed with the patient preoperatively.

Autologous fat grafting is another method for angle or chin augmentation, though results can be unpredictable as fat grafting to highly mimetic areas of the face is often subject to increased resorption and may require serial augmentation. Fat is harvested using standard liposuction techniques, rolled on nonstick gauze pads to process the fat, and is injected along the mandible in a supraperiosteal plane.

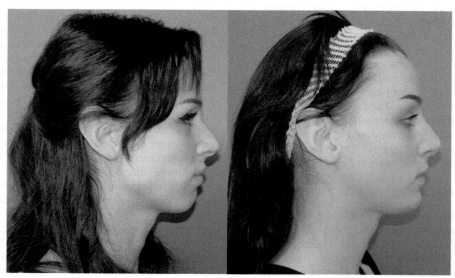

Fig. 12. Preoperative and 1-month postoperative right facial view of the same patient from **Figs. 1–5** after undergoing mandibular angle reduction and advancement and narrowing genioplasty.

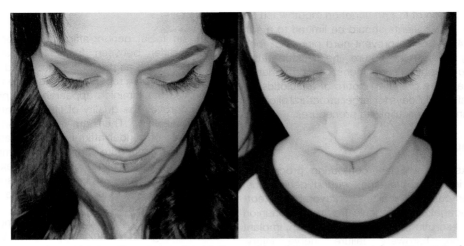

Fig. 13. Preoperative and 1-month postoperative bird's eye view of the same patient from **Figs. 1–5** after undergoing mandibular angle reduction and advancement and narrowing genioplasty.

Genioplasty

Chin masculinization can be performed with alloplastic implants or a bony genioplasty. Implants can aid in accentuating width and sagittal projection but cannot reliably increase the vertical height. Bony genioplasty alternatively can achieve increases in width, height, and projection, though it may need to be supported with interpositional bone grafts for large advancements or lengthening. Implants can either be placed through an intraoral or submental incision.[30]

The intraoral incision should be planned with a wide cuff of mucosa, infiltrated with local anesthesia with epinephrine, and incised down until there is the identification of the mentalis muscle. A large cuff of mentalis muscle should be left to allow for soft tissue and muscle resuspension. The chin is then dissected subperiosteally while protecting the mental nerves. Once adequately exposed, chin implants can be carefully placed and secured to the mandible similar to mandibular angle implants.

The osteotomy for the genioplasty should be designed to achieve the desired changes. To increase the vertical height and projection of the chin, a transverse osteotomy can be designed at least 5 mm below the mental foramen to avoid damage to the inferior alveolar nerve.[31] If the chin needs to be widened, a T-shaped osteotomy should be planned. The authors prefer to use a piezoelectric saw or reciprocating saw for the osteotomy. Any bony gaps in the genioplasty should be filled with autologous bone, bone allograft, or hydroxyapatite granules mixed with blood. The bony segments should be fixated with osteosynthesis material. The wound is thoroughly irrigated with antibiotic irrigation, the mentalis muscle is reapproximated, and the incision is then closed with 3-0 or 4-0 absorbable suture.

POSTOPERATIVE CARE

Lower jaw contouring for gender affirmation can be performed as an outpatient surgery, though patients are often admitted for observation when performed in conjunction with other procedures on the forehead and midface. The largest series on mandibular facial feminization surgery reports that 95% of patients underwent additional feminization procedures, most commonly forehead reconstruction, chondrolaryngoplasty, or rhinoplasty.[19]

Swelling following facial procedures can be significant, so ice packs or controlled cooling therapy are recommended for the first 24 to 48 hours postoperatively.[32] Care must be taken with ice packs to avoid frostbite. Head of bed elevation and compression therapy are also recommended for 6 weeks after surgery which help control edema and assist with soft tissue adaptation to the underlying changes to the neo-mandibular contour. Patients should be counseled that full soft tissue readaptation can take months as there will be initial memory of the soft tissue envelope which may obscure the osseous changes. However, with additive time from surgery, the new mandibular contour will become evident.

As most incisions are within the mouth, excellent oral hygiene is needed to prevent infections. We recommend the use of antiseptic prescription mouthwash for 7 to 10 postoperatively twice daily with salt water rinses after meals. Gentle brushing of teeth can be initiated 48 hours after surgery with a soft bristle toothbrush and over-the-counter mouthwash can be utilized following discontinuation of the prescription mouthwash for 3 weeks. The patients should be limited to a soft diet for 4 weeks, to prevent hard pieces of food pressing through the suture line. Postoperative antibiotic prophylaxis regimens can be variable, but the authors prefer 24 hours of antibiotics for bone grafts and 7 days for larger structural alloplastic implants in masculinizing procedures.

COMPLICATIONS

The risks of lower jaw contouring procedures include infection, bleeding, wound dehiscence, bony contour abnormalities, unfavorable osteotomy propagation, iatrogenic fractures, nonunion or bone resorption, injury to the dentition, implant malposition, hardware failure, nerve injury, "witch's chin" deformity, or soft tissue ptosis.

An infection could manifest as simple cellulitis, abscess, implant infection, or osteomyelitis. Bony contour abnormalities can remodel and resolve over time, and patients should be counseled regarding an initial course of expectant management with close follow-up for persistent concerns. Infection risks are increased with poor dentition, so preoperative dental evaluation and optimization are essential. Preoperative tooth brushing with an antiseptic mouthwash and regular intraoperative antibiotic irrigation may also reduce the risk of infection.

If a genioplasty was performed, numbness of the lower lips and chin from mental or inferior alveolar nerve neuropraxia is common and is often self-limited.[33] Patients can be counseled that sensation should recover as long as there was no nerve transection, however, diminished or altered sensation can persist for up to 9 to 12 months. Older patients are at higher risk for the prolonged recovery of neurosensory function.

"Witch's chin" deformity can occur due to inadequate resuspension of the mentalis muscle, which results in chin soft-tissue ptosis and a tendency toward oral incompetence. Excessive bony reduction during feminizing procedures can result in a loss of support for the overlying facial soft tissues. Iatrogenic jowling can lead to an undesirable result and may require additional surgical treatment, such as a rhytidectomy or neck lift which fall outside of the typical procedures specifically addressing gender dysphoria.[34] Recognition of this has led to some centers counseling patients older than 45 years planning to undergo mandibular border excision exceeding 5 mm that there may be a need for a future face or neck lift surgery.[19]

Most of these complications can be treated nonoperatively and many large series report few complications.[19,35–38]

OUTCOMES

Data on facial gender-affirming surgery significantly differ between facial feminization and masculinization as previously discussed. There is a plethora of data reporting that facial feminization improves the feminine appearance of patients[5,6] and improves the quality of life and patients are highly satisfied.[7] There are fewer reports on the outcomes of gender-affirming facial masculinization as this procedure is much less common due to the highly masculinizing impact of exogenous testosterone. However, small series specifically evaluating facial masculinization have similarly shown high patient satisfaction.[28,29]

Patients seeking facial gender-affirming surgery seek to align their facial appearance with their gender identity and reduce their exposure to social stigma, targeting, and potential interpersonal violence stemming from their morphologic facial gender incongruence. Evidence has shown that facial gender-affirming procedures can be highly effective toward this end. Fisher and colleagues surveyed the public to identify the gender of a patient through a photograph, and facial feminization surgery increased the female gender-typing of these patients from 57% preoperatively to 94% postoperatively.[5] Chen and colleagues performed a study using artificial intelligence and convolutional neural networks to identify the gender of a facial photograph.[6] They found that facial feminization surgery significantly improved the gender-typing of patients when compared to preoperative values.[6]

Ainsworth and Spiegel performed a retrospective study on 247 transfeminine patients in 2010, where 75 underwent facial gender-affirming surgery and 172 did not.[8] They found that transgender women had significantly decreased mental health quality of life compared with the cis-feminine population, though this significantly improved following facial feminization.[8] The same patient-reported outcome tool was used prospectively by Morrison and Capitán in 2020, and they similarly found that facial feminization surgery improved the facial feminization outcome scores in both short term and long term.[7] Additional patient-reported outcome measures have shown significant improvements in anxiety, anger, depression, meaning and purpose, social isolation, and overall positive affect following facial gender-affirming surgery.[39]

SUMMARY

Mandibular contouring is a safe and effective way to masculinize or feminize the face for facial gender-affirming surgery. Facial feminization is largely reductive in nature, aiming to decrease the lower facial width, decrease the chin height, and soften the gonial angle. Facial masculinization is largely additive in nature, with bone grafting or alloplastic augmentation of the mandibular angles and chin. Facial feminization successfully feminizes the face, decreases misgendering, and increases mental health quality of life. Facial masculinization is less common, secondary to the profound masculinizing impact of testosterone.

CLINICS CARE POINTS

- Ensure dental and orthodontic evaluation occurs as part of the preoperative assessment
- Preoperative imaging and virtual planning can be used to augment approaches and identify important structures
- Evaluate facial ptosis prior to reductive procedures to minimize risk of iatrogenic jowling
- Leave healthy cuffs of tissue to sew to during incision planning5) Neuropraxia's are common after lower jaw contouring

SUPPLEMENTARY DATA

Supplementary data related to this article can be found online at https://doi.org/10.1016/j.fsc.2023.04.001.

REFERENCES

1. Ousterhout DK. Feminization of the forehead: Contour changing to improve female aesthetics. Plast Reconstr Surg 1987;79(5):701–11.
2. World Professional Association for Transgender Health. Standards of care for the health of transsexual, transgender, and gender nonconforming people. 7th Edition 2012.
3. JU Berli, Capitán L, Simon D, et al. Facial gender confirmation surgery—review of the literature and recommendations for Version 8 of the WPATH Standards of Care. Int J Transgenderism 2017;18(3):264–70.
4. Coleman E, Bockting W, Botzer M, et al. Standards of Care for the Health of Transsexual, Transgender, and Gender-Nonconforming People, Version 7. Int J Transgenderism 2012;13(4):165–232.
5. Fisher M, Lu SM, Chen K, et al. Facial Feminization Surgery Changes Perception of Patient Gender. Aesthetic Surg J 2020;40(7):703–9.
6. Chen K, Lu SM, Cheng R, et al. Facial Recognition Neural Networks Confirm Success of Facial Feminization Surgery. Plast Reconstr Surg 2020;145(1):203–9.
7. Morrison SD, Capitán-Cañadas F, Sánchez-Garciá A, et al. Prospective Quality-of-Life Outcomes after Facial Feminization Surgery: An International Multicenter Study. Plast Reconstr Surg 2020;145(6):1499–509.
8. Ainsworth TA, Spiegel JH. Quality of life of individuals with and without facial feminization surgery or gender reassignment surgery. Qual Life Res 2010;19(7):1019–24.
9. Coon D, Berli J, Oles N, et al. Facial Gender Surgery: Systematic Review and Evidence-Based Consensus Guidelines from the International Facial Gender Symposium. Plast Reconstr Surg 2022;149(1):212–24.
10. Coleman E, Radix AE, Bouman WP, et al. Standards of Care for the Health of Transgender and Gender Diverse People, Version 8. Int J Transgend Health 2022;23:1–259.
11. Hembree WC, Cohen-Kettenis P, Delemarre-Van De Waal HA, et al. Endocrine treatment of transsexual persons: An endocrine society clinical practice guideline. J Clin Endocrinol Metab 2009;94(9):3132–54.
12. Salibian AA, Bluebond-Langner R. Lip Lift. Facial plastic surgery clinics of North America 2019;27(2):261–6.
13. Antonarakis GS, Kiliaridis S, Scolozzi P. Orientation of the occlusal plane in a Class i adult population. Oral Surgery, Oral Medicine, Oral Pathology and Oral Radiology 2013;116(1):35–40.
14. Ludwig DC, Morrison SD. Should Dental Care Make a Transition? JADA (J Am Dent Assoc) 2018;149(2):79–80.
15. Morrison S, Ettinger RE, Kapadia H, et al. Bimaxillary Surgery with Occlusal Plane Alterations: A New Frontier for Gender Confirmation? Plast Reconstr Surg 2020;146(4):518e–9e.
16. Tawa P, Brault N, Luca-Pozner V, et al. Three-Dimensional Custom-Made Surgical Guides in Facial Feminization Surgery: Prospective Study on Safety and Accuracy. Aesthetic Surg J 2021;41(11):NP1368–78.
17. Gutiérrez-Santamaría J, Simon D, Capitán L, et al. Shaping the lower jaw border with customized cutting guides: development, validation, and application in facial gender-affirming surgery. Facial Plast Surg Aesthet Med 2022. https://doi.org/10.1089/fpsam.2021.0418.
18. Morrison SD, Satterwhite T. Lower Jaw Recontouring in Facial Gender-Affirming Surgery. Facial Plastic Surgery Clinics of North America 2019;27(2):233–42.
19. Simon D, Capitán L, Bailón C, et al. Facial Gender Confirmation Surgery: The Lower Jaw. Description of Surgical Techniques and Presentation of Results. Plast Reconstr Surg 2022;149(4):755e–66e.
20. Zhang C, Ma MW, Xu J-J, et al. Application of the 3D digital ostectomy template (DOT) in mandibular

angle ostectomy (MAO). Journal of cranio-maxillo-facial surgery 2018;46(10):1821–7.

21. Park S, Lee TS. Strategic Considerations for Effective Sagittal Resection of the Mandible to Achieve a Slim and Attractive Jawline. Plast Reconstr Surg 2018;141(1):152–5.

22. Sobol DL, Hopper JS, Ettinger RE, et al. Does the use of a piezoelectric saw improve neurosensory recovery following sagittal split osteotomy? Int J Oral Maxillofac Surg 2022;51(3):371–5.

23. Pavlíková G, Foltán R, Horká M, et al. Piezosurgery in oral and maxillofacial surgery. Int J Oral Maxillofac Surg 2011;40(5):451–7.

24. Altman K. Facial feminization surgery: current state of the art. Int J Oral Maxillofac Surg 2012;41(8): 885–94.

25. Zhang BH, Byrd R, Bradley C, et al. Osseous Genioplasty: Prevention of Witch's Chin Deformity with No-Degloving Technique. Plast Reconstr Surg 2021; 148(5):720e–6e.

26. Jegal JJ, Kang SJ, Kim JW, et al. The utility of a three-dimensional approach with T-shaped osteotomy in osseous genioplasty. Archives of Plastic Surgery 2013;40(4):433–9.

27. Newberry CI, Mobley SR. Chin Augmentation Using Silastic Implants. Facial Plast Surg 2019;35(2): 149–57.

28. Ousterhout DK. Dr. Paul Tessier and facial skeletal masculinization. Ann Plast Surg 2011;67(6):10–5.

29. Deschamps-Braly JC, Sacher CL, Fick J, et al. First Female-to-Male Facial Confirmation Surgery with Description of a New Procedure for Masculinization of the Thyroid Cartilage (Adam's Apple). Plast Reconstr Surg 2017;139(4):883e–7e.

30. Straughan DM, Yaremchuk MJ. Improving Male Chin and Mandible Eesthetics. Clin Plast Surg 2022; 49(2):275–83.

31. Lin HH, Denadai R, Sato N, et al. Avoiding inferior alveolar nerve injury during osseous genioplasty: A guide for the safe zone by three-dimensional virtual imaging. Plast Reconstr Surg 2020;148(2):847–58.

32. Capitán L, Santamaría JG, Simon D, et al. Facial gender confirmation surgery: A protocol for diagnosis, surgical planning, and postoperative management. Plast Reconstr Surg 2020;145(4): 818E–28E.

33. Susarla SM, Ettinger RE, Dodson TB. Is It Necessary to Free the Inferior Alveolar Nerve From the Proximal Segment in the Sagittal Split Osteotomy? J Oral Maxillofac Surg 2020;78(8):1382–8.

34. Rochlin DH, Morrison SD, Harirah M, et al. Face Lift after Facial Feminization Surgery: Indications and Special Considerations. Plast Reconstr Surg 2022; 149(1):107–15.

35. Tirrell AR, Abu El Hawa AA, Bekeny JC, et al. Facial Feminization Surgery: A Systematic Review of Perioperative Surgical Planning and Outcomes. Plastic and Reconstructive Surgery - Global Open 2022; 10(3):E4210.

36. Gupta N, Wulu J, Spiegel JH. Safety of Combined Facial Plastic Procedures Affecting Multiple Planes in a Single Setting in Facial Feminization for Transgender Patients. Aesthetic Plast Surg 2019;43(4): 993–9.

37. Raffaini M, Magri AS, Agostini T. Full Facial Feminization Surgery: Patient Satisfaction Assessment Based on 180 Procedures Involving 33 Consecutive Patients. Plast Reconstr Surg 2016;137(2):438–48.

38. Telang PS. Facial Feminization Surgery: A Review of 220 Consecutive Patients. Indian J Plast Surg 2020; 53(2):244–53.

39. Caprini RM, Oberoi MK, Dejam D, et al. Effect of Gender-affirming Facial Feminization Surgery on Psychosocial Outcomes. Ann Surg 2022. https://doi.org/10.1097/SLA.0000000000005472.

40. Morrison SD, Vyas KS, Motakef S, et al. Facial Feminization: Systematic Review of the Literature. Plast Reconstr Surg 2016;137(6):1759–70.

41. Capitán L, Simon D, Bailón C, et al. The Upper Third in Facial Gender Confirmation Surgery: Forehead and Hairline. J Craniofac Surg 2019;30(5):1393–8.

42. Sedgh J. The Aesthetics of the Upper Face and Brow: Male and Female Differences. Facial Plast Surg 2018;34(2):114–8.

43. Bellinga RJ, Capitán L, Simon D, et al. Technical and clinical considerations for facial feminization surgery with rhinoplasty and related procedures. JAMA Facial Plastic Surgery 2017;19(3):175–81.

44. Ousterhout DK. Mandibular angle augmentation and reduction. Clin Plast Surg 1991;18(1):153–61.

45. Hage JJ, Becking AG, De Graaf FH, et al. Gender-confirming facial surgery: Considerations on the masculinity and femininity of faces. Plast Reconstr Surg 1997;99(7):1799–807.

46. Deschamps-Braly JC. Approach to feminization surgery and facial masculinization surgery: Aesthetic goals and principles of management. J Craniofac Surg 2019;30(5):1352–8.

47. Balaji SM, Balaji P. Square Face Correction by Gonial Angle and Masseter Reduction. Annals of Maxillofacial Surgery 2018;10(1):66–72.

48. Sella-Tunis T, Pokhojaev A, Sarig R, et al. Human mandibular shape is associated with masticatory muscle force. Sci Rep 2018;8(1):6042.

49. Wolfort FG, Parry RG. Laryngeal Chondroplasty for appearance. Plast Reconstr Surg 1975;56(4):371–4.

50. Wolfort FG, Dejerine ES, Ramos DJ, et al. Chondrolaryngoplasty for appearance. Plast Reconstr Surg 1990;86(3):464–9. discussion 470.

Gender Facial Affirmation Surgery: Cheek Augmentation

Brielle Weinstein, MD*, Brandon Alba, MD, Amir Dorafshar, MBChB, Loren Schechter, MD

KEYWORDS

- Cheek augmentation • Facial feminization surgery • Gender affirmation surgery • Lipografting
- Computer-aided design and manufacturing

KEY POINTS

- Understanding anatomy and patient goals guides an individualized surgical plan.
- Commonly used techniques in cheek augmentation include non-autologous filler, lipografting, implants, and zygoma repositioning.
- Cheek augmentation plays an important role in creating facial harmony.

INTRODUCTION

Facial feminization surgery (FFS) represents a constellation of procedures designed to feminize the face of individuals exposed to an androgen puberty.[1] For transgender women seeking social and surgical transition, facial feminization plays an important role in their gender journey. Studies demonstrate improvements in quality of life regarding mental, physical, and social function following FFS.[2] Studies suggest that over one-third of individuals undergo FFS as their first gender-affirming procedure.[3] These useful adjuncts commonly used for rejuvenation may also be used for facial feminization patients.

The cheek, a centrally located structure, influences facial contour in both the anterior and lateral planes. Cheek augmentation uses both surgical and nonsurgical techniques to harmonize facial structures and achieve an overall esthetic result. Techniques may be combined with other facial procedures and include autologous and non-autologous injections, implants, and osseous repositioning. The decision to stage or combine procedures depends on patient goals, operative needs, and surgeon and patient preference. Multiple procedures can be performed safely without an increase in complications.[3] As reported by Chaya and colleagues,[4] satisfaction rates are high with a 3.9% rates of complications.

Recognizing the diversity in the transgender community, it is important to understand the individual's goals and expectations before developing a surgical plan. This article describes a patient-centered approach to facial surgery with a specific consideration given to cheek augmentation.

ANATOMY OF THE CHEEK

Feminine and youthful "cheek bones" colloquially refer to soft tissue fullness at the apex of the cheek. Underlying bony anatomy includes the maxilla inferiorly, inferior orbital rim superiorly, zygoma laterally, and nasal bones medially.[5] As compared with the upper and lower thirds of the face, cephalometric data demonstrate minimal difference between the osseous structures of the midface between cis-females and cis-males.[6] Anatomic differences include a slightly less acute curve of the cis-female orbital rim, less vertical height of the cis-female zygoma, and less bowing of the cis-female zygomatic arch.[7] Soft tissue differences result from exposure to testosterone.[8] The soft tissue of the cis-female cheek is more convex, as compared with the concave shape of the cis-male cheek. In addition, there is more pronounced fullness in the sagittal dimension of the cis-female midface. The fullness of the cis-female midface is due to osseous, fat compartment, and soft tissue variance. The superficial

Division of Plastic and Reconstructive Surgery, Rush University, Affirm: The Rush Center for Gender, Sexuality and Reproductive Health
* Corresponding author. 1725 West Harrison Street, Suite 758, Chicago, IL 60612.
E-mail address: brielle_weinstein@rush.edu

Facial Plast Surg Clin N Am 31 (2023) 393–397
https://doi.org/10.1016/j.fsc.2023.04.002
1064-7406/23/© 2023 Elsevier Inc. All rights reserved.

and deep fat compartments of the cheek are well described in the context of facial aging.[9] They are composed of periorbital fat pads, medial, middle, nasolabial and lateral temporal fat pads, and buccal fat. In patients seeking FFS, these fat compartments can be addressed with rejuvenation procedures as the midface descends and loses volume with age. Owing to forces of gravity, repeated muscular activity, loss of elasticity, and physiologic changes, the midface volume redistributes and descends.

The effects of hormones on facial anatomy have been described using three-dimensional photography and analysis. The cheek (defined as the point where the line between the exocanthion and cheilion and the line between the tragus and alar crest meet) in trans women changed progressively in the transverse and sagittal plans following 3 and 12 months of estrogen use. Specifically, there is lateral deviation in the transverse dimension and an anterior deviation in the sagittal dimension.[8] Skin quality, texture, collagen deposition, and facial hair distribution are also impacted. After 3 to 6 months of estrogen use, the skin softens. After 6 to 12 months, terminal hair growth notably decreases.

Ethnic differences also affect anatomy.[10] In African and East Asian populations, midface projection in the sagittal plane is often decreased as compared with persons of Western European ethnicity. In the coronal plane, African and East Asian populations have increased zygomatic width. Persons of Mediterranean and Western European ethnicity have "narrower" cheeks.[11] During the preoperative consultation, ethnic considerations should be discussed, as these characteristics may influence one's identity and their surgical goals.

PREOPERATIVE PREPARATION

FFS may play an important role in a person's transition, and the medical necessity of FFS is recognized in the updated Standards of Care Version 8 (SOC 8).[12] Before FFS, SOC 8 recommends a single assessment from an appropriate mental or behavioral health provider. Six months of hormone use are recommended so as to allow hormone-related facial changes. If a person does not take hormones, the surgeon should review potential limitations of the overall treatment plan (ie, effect on skin, hair, and subcutaneous fat). Laser or electrolysis may be used for hair removal in the periprocedural period. Recommendations from SOC 8 refer to surgical rather than nonsurgical interventions.

For patients undergoing implant placement and/or osteotomy, computer-assisted technology may be helpful in planning osteotomies and designing custom implants.[13] Not all surgeons elect to use computer-assisted surgery (CAS). If CAS is a component of perioperative planning, discussion of its utility should be part of the shared decision-making process.

TECHNIQUES
Nonsurgical

Non-autologous injectable techniques
Multiple non-autologous injectable materials (aka, "fillers") are available.[14] These vary in permanence, mechanical properties, and composition. Broadly characterized, these "fillers" offer volume replacement and are bio-stimulatory and/or collagen-based. Non-autologous injectables avoid donor site morbidity and may be administered with local or no anesthetic. Injectables can be performed incrementally over time. With the patient awake, they can provide real-time input regarding their esthetic outcome.

Fillers are dependent on rheological properties, such as particle size, G' (firmness and elasticity), cohesivity (ability for the filler to remain in the initial position), concentration of particles, and water uptake.[15] In combination, these characteristics describe the physical response of a filler to applied forces. In the cheek, these forces include pressure of the surrounding tissues, motion from mouth, periorbital movement, and tissue interactions over time. An injector must consider the filler material properties as well as the injection location, volume injected, and plane of injection. Understanding neurovascular midface anatomy, cannula selection, retrograde injection techniques, and small deposition volumes mitigate risk of injection injury.

Hyaluronic acid (HA) preparations offer midface volume replacement and can be selected for certain plane of injection based on rheological properties.[16,17] HA with higher G' is injected in the pre-periosteal plane for medial and lateral malar, submalar, cheek apex and lateral preauricular areas, nasolabial folds in the deep pyriform fossa, and intra-dermally for acne scars. Lower G' fillers can be injected superficially in the subcutaneous plane (ie, mid-cheek accordion lines or nasolabial folds) using a layering technique. HA fillers with an even lower particle size and G' are used in the intradermal or subdermal plane for fine lines and deeper periorbital lines. HA is administered in both deep and superficial planes in the lid-cheek junction. HA injections are temporary, lasting between 6 months and 2 years.

Bio-stimulatory fillers are those that consist of a material that generates a scaffold and inflammatory response, in which new collagen and extracellular matrix are deposited. Examples include calcium hydroxyapatite (CAHA) and poly-l-lactic acid (PLLA). CAHA fillers have an effect for 12 to 18 months, although some studies demonstrate longer effects.[18] Consistent with bio-stimulatory effects, MRI studies by Pavicic and colleagues demonstrate enhancement of soft tissue 2.5 years after injection of CAHA. PLLA stimulates a foreign body response with encapsulation, inflammation, and degradation. In biopsies after PLLA injection, type I and type III collagen are present along with mRNA expression of transforming growth factor (TGF) beta and inhibitors of matrix metalloproteinases.[15]

Complications of fillers include nodules, asymmetry, palpability, and edema. Specific risks of HA in the periorbital region include the Tyndall effect, a blue hue related to light scattering in water particles.[19] If vascular compromise occurs, hyaluronidase can be injected into the affected area with adjunctive treatments. The receipt of illicit subcutaneous injections is more common in trans women.[20] At times, these substances may be non-Federal Drug Administration approved or even nonmedical grade substances such as liquid silicone, mineral oil, biopolymer, or collagen. As a gender-affirming provider, it is important to counsel patients on the importance of using a qualified provider, approved materials, and medical risks associated with filler use.

Surgical

FFS includes a constellation of surgical procedures, which can include cheek augmentation. A National Surgical Quality Improvement Program database demonstrated that 11.7% of patients undergoing FFS have cheek augmentation included.[4] In a systematic review with 4108 patients over 18 studies, zygoma augmentation was performed in 13.9% of facial feminization patients, zygoma osteotomy in 0.3%, and midface lift in 0.4%.[21] Nearly half of the patients were underwent surgery on an ambulatory basis.[4]

Fat grafting
Liposuction and fat grafting to the midface provide long-lasting autologous volume addition without the morbidity of other more invasive surgical techniques.[22] Goals of facial fat grafting typically include a smooth lid-cheek junction, an increased convexity of the medial and lateral cheek, and amelioration of the nasolabial fold. Whether in combination with other surgical procedures or performed in isolation, lipografting involves fat harvest, typically with tumescent fluid and cannula, fat processing, and injections, typically with cannula.

Fat grafting to the face is considered a safe procedure with a low-risk profile. Rare complications include bleeding, infection, reactions to local or general anesthesia, and unfavorable esthetic results.

Each step in the process affects graft take.[23] Recommendations for fat harvest include the use of 3 to 4 mm cannula. The location of harvest has not been demonstrated to affect graft take. The goals of fat preparation include separating the adipocytes from serum, blood, damaged cells, and infiltrate. Options for fat preparation include centrifugation, gauze rolling, and filtration. Injection is optimized with a 2 to 2.5 mm cannula deposited in small aliquots with a low-shear stress environment.[24] Long-term results of fat grafting differ depending on the vascularity of the wound bed.

Fat placement in the deep medial fat pad aids in projection and effacement of nasolabial folds.[25] Studies demonstrate an increase of 1.92 ± 0.26 times the height ($P < 0.01$) of the medial cheek when injected into multiple fat pads.[26] Cohen and colleagues[27] advocated for injection into the buccal fat pad with up to 2.7cc of fat. In one study, a mean of 29.3cc of fat was injected per cheek with a 27.1% cheek volume increase at 12 months.[28]

Alloplastic implant cheek augmentation
Malar implants provide an alternative approach to treating the midface especially in patients with a negative cheek vector. A lack of projection of the bony anatomy can contribute to accelerated descent and age-related changes of the midface.[29] Age-related bony changes include the loss of volume at the pyriform region of the nose and the inferior and lateral aspects of the orbital rim.[5] A midface implant can be used to address volume loss of the infraorbital region as well as augment the tear through and provide support for the lower eyelid. By supporting the midmalar tissue, the implant fills the nasolabial fold and reduces the prominence of the nose.[30] Implants may be helpful in cases of an under developed and under projected zygoma with adequate bizygomatic width.[13]

The two most common types of implants used in cheek augmentation include silicone and porous polyethylene (PPE).[31] Silicone implants can be placed through smaller incisions, are customizable at the time of surgery, and can be easily removed. Risks include encapsulation and malposition. PPE creates a more permanent construct with tissue integration and individualization. As a result of tissue integration, PPE implants are more difficult to remove.

Implants are placed through either periorbital incisions or intraoral incisions within the maxillary vestibule.[31] Dissection is performed in the subperiosteal plane over the malar region and the anterior portion of the zygomatic arch. Over-dissection should be avoided as an excessively large pocket can contribute to implant mobility. Implant placement abutting the infraorbital neurovascular bundle should also be avoided.

As with all implants, malar implants pose risks of infection and extrusion. Postoperative swelling is not uncommon, and patients should be monitored closely for hematoma formation. Patients should also be counseled that in the immediate postoperative period, swelling and disruption of the local musculature can cause abnormal animation during facial expressions; this is typically temporary and subsides within 1 to 2 weeks.[31] Despite fixation, implant malposition may occur. Issues such as implant malposition and asymmetry may require implant removal and/or repositioning. Implants may be suitable in patients for whom support of the midface tissues is warranted and unable to be accomplished with injectable materials alone.

Zygoma osteotomy

For some patients, osseous craniofacial reconstruction involving zygoma osteotomy and repositioning may be required. The results are long lasting and provide soft tissue support through the aging process. Proponents of midface osteotomies note that although this method is more technically difficult than implant placement, filler, or fat grafting, osteotomies are a more permanent solution, which are less likely to require future revisions.[32]

Surgical exposure can be achieved through maxillary vestibular and preauricular incisions. Planning may include computer-aided design/computer-aided manufacturing (CAD/CAM) design of operative guides. These are placed at planned osteotomy sites, and the jig can be placed through a maxillary vestibular and small preauricular incision. Reduction with titanium plates and predrilled pilot holes allows for symmetric and reproducible results.[13] Generally, the zygoma is moved medially and inferior to give a more feminized and convex cheek. Other techniques for osteotomy include movement of the zygomatic malar complex with a segmentalized zygoma osteotomy. This requires exposure through a coronal incision, intra-oral and trans-conjunctival incisions.[32] Zygoma osteotomy can pose risks of contour irregularity, trismus, palpable step off, and hardware-related complication.

SUMMARY

Cheek augmentation plays an important role in creating facial harmony during feminizing facial procedures.[30,33,34] A variety of surgical and nonsurgical techniques are available, each with their own risk–benefit profile.[35] Attention to patient-specific cheek anatomy, including ethnic and age considerations, is warranted. As gender-affirming surgeons look toward the future, surgeons should anticipate an increasing incidence of FFS procedures to include cheek augmentation. Surgeons should be attentive to patient goals and familiar with a range of surgical and nonsurgical modalities.[36]

CLINICS CARE POINTS

- Attention to the midface is critical to harmonize the cheeks with the rest of the face and should be included in comprehensive facial feminization surgery.
- A patient-centered approach to selection of the optimal technique includes discussion of patient goals and coordination with multidisciplinary team.
- Techniques offered to the patient may among nonsurgical and surgical treatment plans based on risk profile and patient goals.

DISCLOSURE

Dr L. Schechter has disclosures for book royalties from Springer and Elsevier publishing.

REFERENCES

1. Dechamps-Braly JC. Facial gender confirmation surgery facial feminization surgery and facial masculinization surgery. In: Schechter LS, editor. Gender confirmation surgery. Switzerland: Springer International Publishing; 2020. p. 323–31. essay.
2. Ainsworth TA, Spiegel JH. Quality of life of individuals with and without facial feminization surgery or gender reassignment surgery. Qual Life Res 2010; 19:1019–24.
3. Chaya BF, Boczar D, Rodriguez Colon R, et al. Comparative outcomes of partial and full facial feminization surgery: a retrospective cohort study. J Craniofac Surg 2021;32(7):2397–400.
4. Chaya BF, Berman ZP, Boczar D, et al. Current trends in facial feminization surgery: an assessment of safety and style. J Craniofac Surg 2021;32(7): 2366–9.
5. Mendelson B, Wong C-H. Changes in the facial skeleton with aging: implications and clinical applications in facial rejuvenation. Aesthetic Plast Surg 2012;36(4):756.

6. Frey ST. New diagnostic tenet of the esthetic mid-face for clinical assessment of anterior malar projection. Angle Orthod 2013;83:790–4.

7. Schlager S, Rüdell A. Sexual dimorphism and population affinity in the human zygomatic structure—comparing surface to outline data. Anat Rec 2017;300:226–37.

8. Tebbens M, Nota NM, Liberton NPTJ, et al. Gender-affirming hormone treatment induces facial feminization in transwomen and masculinization in transmen: quantification by 3D scanning and patient-reported outcome measures. J Sex Med 2019;16(5):746–54.

9. Gierloff M, Stöhring C, Buder T, et al. Aging changes of the midfacial fat compartments: a computed tomographic study. Plast Reconstr Surg 2012;129(1):263.

10. Saad A, Hewett S, Nolte M, et al. Ethnic rhinoplasty in female patients: the neoclassical canons revisited. Aesthetic Plast Surg 2018;42(2):565–76.

11. Nasal analysis: considerations for ethnic variation. Villanueva, nathaniel; afrooz, paul; carboy, jourdan; rohrich, rod. Plast Reconstr Surg 2019;143(6):1179e–88e.

12. Coleman E, Radix AE, Bouman WP, et al. Standards of care for the health of transgender and gender diverse people, version 8. International Journal of Transgender Health 2022;23(sup1):S1–259.

13. Louis M, Qiu CS, Travieso R, et al. Computer-aided planning and execution in facial gender surgery: approaches, concepts, and implementation. Plastic and Reconstructive Surgery - Global Open 2022;10(5):e4330.

14. Sarah Crowley J, Kream E, Fabi S, et al. Facial rejuvenation with fat grafting and fillers. Aesthetic Surg J 2021;41(Issue Supplement_1):S31–8.

15. Hee CK, Shumate GT, Narurkar V, et al. Rheological properties and in vivo performance characteristics of soft tissue fillers. Dermatol Surg 2015;41(Suppl 1):S373–81.

16. Goodman GJ, Swift A, Remington B, et al. Current concepts in the use of voluma, volift, and volbella. Plast Reconstr Surg 2015;136(Issue 5S):139S–48S.

17. Mckee D, Remington K, Swift A, et al. Effective rejuvenation with hyaluronic acid fillers: current advanced concepts. Plast Reconstr Surg 2019;143(6):1277e–89e.

18. Pavicic T. Complete biodegradable nature of calcium hydroxylapatite after injection for malar enhancement: an MRI study. Clin Cosmet Investig Dermatol 2015;8:19–25.

19. Wang Y, Massry G, Holds JB. Complications of periocular dermal fillers. Facial Plast Surg Clin North Am 2021;29(2):349–57.

20. Sergi FD, Wilson EC. Filler use among trans women: correlates of feminizing subcutaneous injections and their health consequences. Transgend Health 2021;6(2):82–90.

21. Tirrell AR, Abu El H, Areeg A, et al. Facial feminization surgery: a systematic review of perioperative surgical planning and outcomes. Plastic and Reconstructive Surgery - Global Open 2022;10(3):e4210.

22. Safa B, Lin W, Salim A, et al. Current concepts in feminizing gender surgery. Plast Reconstr Surg 2019;143(5):1081e–91e.

23. Gutowski KA, ASPS Fat Graft Task Force. Current applications and safety of autologous fat grafts: a report of the ASPS fat graft task force. Plast Reconstr Surg 2009;124(1):272–80.

24. Zielins ER, Brett EA, Longaker MT, et al. Autologous fat grafting: the science behind the surgery. Aesthet Surg J 2016;36(4):488–96.

25. Rohrich RJ, Pessa JE, Ristow B. The youthful cheek and the deep medial fat compartment. Plast Reconstr Surg 2008;121(6):2107.

26. Sheng L, Yu Z, Li S, et al. Midface Rejuvenation With Autologous Fat Grafting. J Craniofac Surg 2022. https://doi.org/10.1097/SCS.0000000000008949. Epub ahead of print. PMID: 36000767.

27. Cohen SR, Fireman E, Hewett S, et al. Buccal fat pad augmentation for facial rejuvenation. Plast Reconstr Surg 2017;139(6):1273e.

28. Wang W, Xie Y, Huang RL, et al. Facial contouring by targeted restoration of facial fat compartment volume: the midface. Plast Reconstr Surg 2017;139(3):563–72.

29. Binder WJ, Azizzadeh B. Malar and submalar augmentation. Facial Plast Surg Clin North Am 2008;16(1):11–32, v.

30. Raffaini M, Magri AS, Agostini T. Full facial feminization surgery: patient satisfaction assessment based on 180 procedures involving 33 consecutive patients. Plast Reconstr Surg 2016;137(2):438–48.

31. Niamtu J 3rd. Essentials of cheek and midface implants. J Oral Maxillofac Surg 2010;68(6):1420–9. Epub 2010 Apr 9. PMID: 20381942.

32. Lundgren TK, Farnebo F. Midface osteotomies for feminization of the facial skeleton. Plast Reconstr Surg Glob Open 2017;5(1):e1210.

33. Morrison SD, Vyas KS, Motakef S, et al. Facial feminization: systematic review of the literature. Plast Reconstr Surg 2016;137(6):1759–70.

34. Whitehead DM, Schechter LS. Cheek augmentation techniques. Facial Plast Surg Clin North Am 2019;27(2):199–206.

35. Jumaily JS. Cheek augmentation in gender-affirming facial surgery. Otolaryngol Clin North Am 2022. https://doi.org/10.1016/j.otc.2022.05.004. S0030-6665(22)00061-00065.

36. MacGregor JL, Chang YC. Minimally invasive procedures for gender affirmation. Dermatol Clin 2020;38(2):249–60.

Injectable Treatments and Nonsurgical Aspects of Gender Affirmation

Grace T. Wu, MD[a], Anni Wong, MD[a], Jason D. Bloom, MD[a,b],*

KEYWORDS

• Facial gender affirmation • Facial feminization • Transgender • Botulinum toxin • Dermal filler

KEY POINTS

- Transgender people in the United States are more likely than the general population to be impoverished, and thus the cost of injectables may be a more salient concern. Providers should be able to counsel patients about surgical options, the cost of which may be covered by health insurance.
- There is overlap in what is considered beautiful in masculine and feminine faces. Not all beautification measures will contribute to correct gendering in a transgender person.
- Feminizing the nose and mandible are reductive procedures and unlikely to be achieved through nonsurgical means alone.
- As stand-alone procedures, injectables are unlikely to meet expectations, particularly in trans women. However, injectables are still a valuable tool to be considered in those seeking facial gender-affirming treatments.

INTRODUCTION

There has been an increasing amount of literature available on facial gender affirmation surgery in recent years; however, there remains a paucity of literature available on nonsurgical treatments, in particular, injectable treatments for facial gender affirmation. A 2019 review describes the current landscape.[1]

Nonsurgical treatments are less invasive and capable of more subtle and precise changes in appearance. They are usually reversible and have a smaller upfront cost; however, they may require multiple treatments for the best results. This may be an opportunity for an individual to "try-out" more masculine or feminine features to see if they want to continue with a more permanent surgery in the future. As a stand-alone procedure or an adjunct to hormone and/or surgical therapy, nonsurgical treatments can help to fine-tune facial features to one's satisfaction.

Nonsurgical options include injectable treatments such as neurotoxin and dermal filler, laser or electrolysis, and minimally invasive procedures, such as thread lifts and energy-based skin-tightening devices. This article focuses on injectable treatments for the upper, middle, and lower thirds of the face (Table 1).

Facial Feminization Versus Masculinization

Trans women are more likely to seek facial gender-affirming care than trans men.[2] This is likely because the virilizing effects of endogenous testosterone on the face and body are variably reversed by estrogen therapy and gonadotropin-releasing hormone analog therapy. This is true particularly for bony changes of the face—frontal bossing and mandibular enlargement will not be affected by hormone therapy, and unfortunately, these facial features can be quite telling of an individual's assigned sex at birth. Facial fat distribution will

a Department of Otorhinolaryngology, University of Pennsylvania, 3737 Market Street, Suite 302, Philadelphia, PA 19104, USA; b Bloom Facial Plastic Surgery, Two Town Place, Suite 110, Bryn Mawr, PA 19010, USA
* Corresponding author.
E-mail address: drjbloom@bloomfps.com

Facial Plast Surg Clin N Am 31 (2023) 399–406
https://doi.org/10.1016/j.fsc.2023.04.004
1064-7406/23/© 2023 Elsevier Inc. All rights reserved.

Table 1
Nonsurgical methods of gender affirmation

	Feminizing	Masculinizing
Upper third	Filler • Supraorbital ridge • Temporal hollows Botulinum toxin • Frontalis (for horizontal forehead lines and changing brow position) • Procerus and corrugators (for glabellar lines and to raise medial brow) • Orbicularis oculi (to raise lateral brow) Other • Eyebrow depilation • Microblading	Other • Eyebrow depilation • Microblading
Middle third	Filler • Midface/cheeks Botulinum toxin • Inferior orbicularis oculi (for eye aperture widening)	Filler • Midface/cheeks (may not be beneficial for all)
Lower third	Filler • Pogonion • Lips Botulinum toxin • Masseters (to induce muscle atrophy and lower face narrowing) • Orbicularis oris (to evert vermillion border) Other • Laser hair removal	Filler • Mandibular border

change along with body fat distribution, but many trans women on hormone therapy will still seek facial feminization procedures.

For purposes of clarity, the discussion of gender affirmation in this article will be limited to transgender individuals who are interested in binary male-to-female or female-to-male transitions, particularly those who are looking to assimilate to a binary esthetic standard in terms of their facial appearance, an experience of "transness" that is by no means representative of the many transgender experiences that exist. The facial alterations suggested will adhere to classic Western esthetics in terms of how facial features contribute to gendering. The literature available on facial gender affirmation surgery and facial sexual dimorphism reveals ambiguity regarding the crossover and considerable overlap in what is considered attractive in both men and women. This gray area between gendering and beautification measures begs further investigation.

History of Injectables for Transgender Patients

A unique aspect of injectables for transgender people is the history of transgender women

seeking fillers for body contouring and facial feminization by nonmedical providers, sometimes in group settings called "pumping parties."[3] For transgender women, facial feminization and body contouring are not just esthetic procedures. Such treatments alleviate gender dysphoria and make it possible for them to pass through society as cisgender women, enabling them to more easily obtain employment and avoid discrimination and harassment. Silicone is often used in the aforementioned informal settings; however, decades of clinician experience with injectable silicone, dating back to the 1960s when it was undergoing Food and Drug Administration (FDA)-regulated clinical investigation for soft tissue augmentation,[4] have shown it to be fraught with complications. Silicone is not an acceptable esthetic injection material.

Nevertheless, people continue to seek out liquid silicone from nonmedical providers. According to a cross-sectional survey of 631 trans women conducted in the San Francisco Bay Area from 2016 to 2017, about 5% had received filler from someone who was not a medical professional.[5] It is very likely that the cost differential is a major determinant. The 2015 US Transgender

Survey found that nearly a third of respondents were living in poverty compared with 12% of the US population. In the year before completing the survey, 33% of respondents did not go to a health care provider when needed because they could not afford it.[6]

Candidates for Injectables for Gender Affirmation

According to the World Professional Association for Transgender Health, Standards of Care Version 8, in order to access gender-affirming medical and surgical therapy, a transgender person's gender incongruence must be marked and sustained. This should be determined by a health care practitioner with a master's degree or equivalent training in a clinical field relevant to the role.[7] However, men are increasingly seeking injectable treatments, such as botulinum toxin and facial fillers.[8,9] There is no such requirement that cisgender people seek an approval letter to receive esthetic treatments. Therefore, there currently exists a contradiction. Is it ethical to provide feminizing or masculinizing injectable treatments to transgender individuals, particularly fully reversible treatments, without a supporting letter from a qualified health care practitioner? In certain situations, the answer is probably yes.

As we are considering a less invasive, and often fully reversible, alternative to surgery, a standard informed consent process should be adequate. When in doubt, or when the changes desired are extreme, unusual or permanent, a supporting letter should be obtained. A discussion of ethics beyond the aforementioned situation is beyond the scope of this clinical technique-focused article. The authors recommend that a thorough informed consent is obtained before performing any gender-affirmation treatment.

ANATOMIC FACIAL AREAS
Upper Third

There are varying opinions on which third of the face most contributes to facial gender recognition. Ousterhout, who pioneered surgical forehead feminization in the 1980s, believed that it was the upper third, including the nasofrontal angle.[10] Perhaps the closest we come to a scientific investigation of this question is the 2011 survey by Spiegel, in which he found that the forehead has the most significant impact in determining gender of a patient.[11]

The upper third of the face, from trichion to glabella, contains numerous features that suggest one's assigned sex at birth. Aside from the hairline, the suprabrow ridge and eyebrow orientation are perhaps most signifying of one's assigned sex at birth. Less prominent factors include temple contour and depth of forehead and glabellar rhytids. Injectables can alter many of these facial issues.

Forehead

A smooth and gently convex forehead without a suprabrow ridge or frontal bossing conveys femininity, whereas a forehead with a prominent suprabrow ridge and frontal bossing reads as masculine. In trans women, filler can be used to smooth the contour of the forehead and create a more gentle convex shape. When injecting filler for this purpose, a precise knowledge of the anatomy of the supratrochlear, supraorbital, and temporal arteries is paramount. Aspiration is recommended before injecting. Filler can be injected via a serial puncture technique using a needle down to the level of the bone at evenly spaced points above the suprabrow ridge or there can be a single lateral entry point using a cannula to address the right and left sides of the forehead. Filler should be deposited supraperiosteally to avoid intra-arterial injection. Belotero Volume[12] and Juvederm Voluma[13] have been used to contour the forehead. The amount used is variable and ranges up to about 3cc.[13] Individuals with very prominent frontal bossing should be advised that filler may only provide minimal improvement in appearance and that surgery would produce better results.

Botulinum toxin for frontalis muscle denervation to prevent horizontal forehead rhytids should also be performed for full forehead feminization. A 2013 study of Japanese men and women found that men have increased forehead wrinkles in all age groups,[14] which suggests that effacing horizontal forehead wrinkles may result in a more feminine forehead. Trans women with receding hairlines will generally require a wider and higher injection pattern of the frontalis muscle than ciswomen. In any individual with temporal tuft recession (ie, a norwood 3 hairline), the treatment should extend into these areas to prevent unnatural wrinkling in the temporal region.[15] Aside from the higher dosage required to treat a larger surface area, as cisgender men require higher dosages of botulinum toxin than cisgender women,[16] trans women may also require higher dosages per injection site. Static wrinkles still present after botulinum toxin therapy can be treated with intradermal filler injection.

Eyebrows

The feminine eyebrow has a peak between the lateral limbus and the lateral canthus, and the lateral portion sits above the orbital rim. The masculine eyebrow is flat and lies lower, along the orbital rim.

It is prudent not to forget that selective eyebrow depilation can be an effective option for certain individuals with favorable eyebrows (ie, eyebrows in which an arch may be created or minimized with or without the aid of an eyebrow pencil). As cost may be of concern for transgender individuals, patients should be made aware of any low-cost alternatives of improving brow esthetics. Microblading, a tattoo technique in which feather-like strokes create realistic looking brows, can be considered for those with sparse eyebrow hair as an alternative to using an eyebrow pencil. An alternative to microblading is hair transplantation to the eyebrows, which should be sought with an experienced hair transplant surgeon.

Botulinum toxin is commonly used to alter the position of the eyebrows. It may be used to lift or depress the brow. Applying botulinum toxin to the glabellar complex, including the procerus and corrugator muscles, lifts the medial brow. A randomized double-blind trial of 80 men found that a dosage double that would be used on most women was more efficacious and durable.[17] Based on this study, trans women may also benefit from significantly higher dosages in the glabella.

Selective application in 1-3 Botox equivalent units to the orbicularis oculi muscle underneath the lateral brow will allow the lateral brow to lift as well.[18] The judicious use of botulinum toxin in the frontalis muscle, making sure not to administer it lateral to the brow peak or lateral limbus, can enhance the appearance of the brow arch. On the other hand, in transgender men, forehead treatment should extend past the brow peak and laterally enough to prevent eyebrow arching. Botulinum toxin can be used to flatten the brow by injecting it into the inferior portion of the frontalis muscle, just above the peak of the eyebrow. Again, transgender women may require higher dosages than cisgender women. The opposite may be true for transgender men.

Temples

The temple should be flat or slightly convex on anterior view of the feminine face. Cisgender adult men tend to have a slightly concave temporal region. When re-volumizing the temple, efforts should be focused on the anterior aspect outside of the hairline and below the temporal fusion line. Injecting more posteriorly has minimal effect on appearance and tends to be a waste of product. The structures to be concerned about when addressing temple hollowing are the temporal branch of the facial nerve and the superficial, middle, and deep temporal vessels. There are no fillers

that are FDA-approved for volumization of the temples. The use of Juvederm Voluma, Juvederm Ultra Plus,[18] and Restylane[19] has all been reported. Higher G′ products are preferable for use in this area.[20] Both hyaluronic acid (HA) and calcium hydroxyapatite fillers have been safely used to volumize the temple. Initial injection volumes for mild hollowing range between 1 and 2cc per side.[19,21] When injecting, the superficial temporal artery should be palpated, identified, and avoided.

Middle Third

The middle third of the face, from glabella to subnasale, includes the eyes, cheeks, and nose. The nose likely plays the biggest role in determining gender given its prominence and central location on the face. An experiment by Chronicle and colleagues[22] found that participants were more likely than not to be able to correctly guess someone's gender based on the nose alone in oblique or profile views.

Nose

The nose is the most complex area to address and injectables are unlikely to adequately feminize a large, masculine looking nose. By nature, injectables can only serve to augment the nose, and so achieving soft femininity of the nose is difficult with filler. Therefore, a trans woman with an overprojected nose and a large dorsal hump has limited options when it comes to injectable filler for the nose, also known as liquid or injectable rhinoplasty.

Smaller and less projected than masculine noses, feminine noses are characterized by a straighter or slightly sloped dorsum, a larger nasofrontal and nasolabial angle, and a narrower tip. On profile view, the radix should be located between the supratarsal crease and the upper lid margin. A common maneuver with liquid rhinoplasty is dorsal nasal hump camouflage, however, whether this actually feminizes the nose is unclear. In an already overprojected nose, camouflaging a hump by administering filler superior to the hump may unnaturally lengthen the nose, a tradeoff that is acceptable for certain individuals. Although the nose may be more aesthetically pleasing, it is unclear if liquid rhinoplasty would contribute to an individual's correct gender identification.

Owing to cost, transience of effect and uncertain efficacy in correct gender identification, the authors recommend surgical rhinoplasty over liquid rhinoplasty in most transfeminine individuals seeking feminizing rhinoplasty.

Eyes

Larger eyes are considered more feminine and botulinum toxin can be used to widen the eye aperture, as demonstrated by Flynn and colleagues[23] who performed a case series with 15 women, injecting crow's feet with 12 units of Botox and the pretarsal inferior orbicularis oculi muscle with 2 units. The injection in the pretarsal orbicularis oculi muscle is just subdermal in the midpupillary line, about 2–3 mm below the ciliary margin. In order to avoid inadvertently inducing ectropion, it is important not to perform this maneuver in individuals with a delayed lower lid snap test or preexisting scleral show.

Cheeks

Feminine cheeks are characterized as round and full, whereas masculine cheeks are characterized as flat and angular. Fullness in the cheeks can readily be produced using filler. Restylane Lyft, Restylane Contour, and Juvederm Voluma XC have FDA approval to be used in the midface. Radiesse (+) is also commonly used to enhance the midface, though it is not FDA-approved for this purpose. HA and calcium hydroxyapatite fillers should first be injected more deeply onto the bone and into the deep facial fat compartments followed by a layered injection, usually with a cannula, to produce volume in the more superficial fat pads of the face. Product is injected in the cheeks at multiple different layers including, the subdermal, subcutaneous, and supraperiosteal levels. Amounts ranging from 1 to 3cc per side have been reported with higher volumes injected for greater cheek volume loss.[24]

Lower Third

The lower third of the face, from subnasale to menton, has masculine and feminine features, most notably the size and shape of the mandible and chin, and the presence of facial hair.

Mandible and jawline

The male mandible is wider, taller, and has increased lateral flare at the gonial angles. The increased height is perhaps most prominent at the chin. Anthropological studies have identified more well-developed lateral tubercles in male mandibles which contribute to the broad, square appearance of the chin.[25] A common standard used is that the width of the chin is equal to the width of the nasal base in females, whereas it is equal to the width of the mouth in males. Males also have greater muscular bulk than females, and this is evident in the masseter muscle which contributes to the width of the lower face.

As is the case with rhinoplasty, feminizing the male mandible is a reductive procedure and difficult to fully achieve with injectables alone. The greatest change can be obtained with neurotoxin administration to the masseter muscle, which can produce dramatic lower face narrowing by inducing atrophy of that muscle. Botulinum toxin to the masseter muscle should be injected into the inferior aspect of the muscle, which is its bulkiest part. The soft tissue in this area can be thick, and it is important to make sure to use a needle of adequate length to reach the masseter muscle. It can be helpful to have the patient bite down on their back teeth so that it is easier to palpate the muscle when injecting. Care should be taken not to inject too anterosuperiorly, which may chemodeinnervate the risorius leading to an asymmetric smile. A review of studies investigating botulinum toxin for masseter muscle hypertrophy found that doses used ranged from 20 to 56 Botox equivalent units using onabotulinum toxin A or abobotulinum toxin A.[26]

The increased height of the mandible in the trans woman is impossible to disguise using injectables. However, some trans women may benefit from filler administration to the pogonion to create a more pointed chin. By augmenting the chin at the pogonion, it actually gives the appearance of a narrowed lower third of the face in the anterior view. This should only be done for appropriate candidates and those who do not already have an overprojected pogonion. Botulinum toxin administration to the mentalis muscle may decrease anterior projection of the chin, but it may also flatten the anterior chin, making it appear broader. Trans women with tall and wide mandibles should be advised that surgery would best serve to feminize their mandibles.

Masculinization of the jawline to achieve a more prominent and angular lower part of the face can be attempted with filler augmentation. Juvederm Volux is the newest filler that is FDA-approved to improve jawline definition and was released in the United States in 2022. Radiesse (+) also has an FDA jawline indication and is another good choice for the mandible because of its strength and very high G'. Before the release of this new product, clinicians typically used products such as Restylane Lyft or Juvederm Voluma. Filler strategically distributed at points from the midline to the gonial angle can help produce a broader, strongly supported lower face.[27] Filler should be deposited supraperiosteally or in the deep subcutaneous tissue. One should be cognizant of and avoid damaging the facial artery, which runs near the anterior border of the masseter muscle and crosses over the mandible at the antegonial notch. It can easily be palpated with its strong pulse and avoided.

Lips

Feminine lips differ from masculine lips in many ways. Women have greater vermillion show in both the upper and the lower lips, but the total length of the upper lip is shorter in women than in men. In addition, feminine lips are characterized by greater anterior projection of the vermillion of the upper and lower lips. In both genders, the upper lip should have less volume and vermillion show than the lower lip. Common techniques for lip augmentation include outlining the vermillion to highlight it and vertical tenting to increase volume and provide more red lip show. Of note, it is important not to inject past the wet–dry border of the lip and to place the filler in the submucosal layer, superficial to the orbicularis oris muscle. When performing lip augmentation, HA fillers are preferred. Revanesse Versa Lips, Juvederm Ultra, Juvederm Volbella, Restylane-L, and Restylane Kysse are all FDA-approved for lip augmentation.

A trending procedure called the "lip flip" uses botulinum toxin injected into the orbicularis oris muscle of the upper or lower lip to paralyze that portion of the muscle to cause eversion of the red lip. Injections are placed about 2 mm superior or inferior to the vermillion border, and around four injection sites should be planned.[28]

Facial hair

For the transgender patient, the presence or absence of hair plays a crucial role in the affirmation of gender and subsequently their self-confidence and self-identity in society. A survey of transgender and nonbinary individuals revealed that of those surveyed who had sought facial treatments, the most common procedure obtained was laser hair removal (LHR).[29]

The presence of facial hair in the lower and lateral face is a strong indicator of a masculine gender. Treatments for hair removal range from temporary methods such as shaving, waxing, tweezing, and depilatory creams to more permanent methods such as LHR and electrolysis. Hair removal can be performed via Nd:YAG, diode, alexandrite or ruby laser, or intense pulsed light.[30] Multiple sessions are often needed to achieve the desired hair reduction. As LHR uses light waves at various frequencies to target melanin in the hair shaft, a high melanin gradient between skin and hair follicles is necessary to achieve optimal results. Individuals with light hair and light skin desiring hair removal can use electrolysis, in which each hair follicle is treated individually using a needle inserted into the hair follicle. Electrolysis also requires multiple sessions and is often more painful than laser therapies.

SUMMARY

There are numerous areas in the face that can be made more feminine or masculine using injectables. Features in the upper third of the face, particularly the forehead contour and brow position are likely to contribute most to correct gender identification. Other prominent features in the face such as the nose and the mandible also contribute to an individual's facial femininity or masculinity. However, whether or not feminization of isolated facial features or a partial feminization through injectables allows for correct gender identification in the real world is unknown.

An important consideration to keep in mind when seeing transgender patients is that many injectable treatments may be seen as cost-prohibitive. There is progress in the realm of insurance companies covering gender affirmation care, but the coverage for facial gender affirmation surgery is sparse and almost nothing for facial injectables treatment. Any clinician who offers injectables for transgender patients should be aware of surgical treatments for facial gender affirmation to guide the patient to the treatment that best suits their needs and budget. In addition, patients should be strongly cautioned against seeking out unlicensed treatments for facial feminization or body contouring.

As a stand-alone procedure for facial gender affirmation, particularly in trans women, injectables are likely to fall short of meeting expectations. Nevertheless, injectables have a role in the gender affirmation of transgender patients. They can be a valuable tool for the patient who is transitioning but unsure of whether or not they want to proceed with definitive surgery, or they can allow a patient to fine-tune their appearance after facial gender affirmation surgery.

CLINICS CARE POINTS

- Frontal bossing, supraorbital ridges, and eyebrow orientation can be feminized using filler and neurotoxin.

- Masculine noses will benefit more from surgical rhinoplasty rather than liquid rhinoplasty, since feminization of the nose is a reductive procedure that cannot be achieved with filler.

- Filler can readily produce full, feminine cheeks. Several fillers are FDA-approved for use in the midface.

- Lip filler is an effective treatment to feminize the lips. HA fillers are preferred for use in the lips.

- Certain differences between male and female mandibles cannot be disguised using injectables, and surgery may be the ideal treatment in many transfeminine dividuals. However, neurotoxin can produce a dramatic narrowing of the lower face when injected in the masseter muscle.

DISCLOSURES

Dr J.D. Bloom is a consultant, advisory board member, speaker's bureau member, trainer, and clinical investigator for Galderma and Allergan. He is also a consultant, advisory board member, speaker's bureau member, and trainer for Revance Therapeutics and Endo Aesthetics.

REFERENCES

1. Ascha M, Swanson MA, Massie JP, et al. Nonsurgical management of facial masculinization and feminization. Aesthet Surg J 2019;39(5):NP123–37.
2. Ginsberg BA, Calderon M, Seminara NM, et al. A potential role for the dermatologist in the physical transformation of transgender people: a survey of attitudes and practices within the transgender community. J Am Acad Dermatol 2016;74:303–8.
3. Nett, Dani. For Trans Women, Silicone 'Pumping' Can Be A Blessing And A Curse. National Public Radio. Available at: https://www.npr.org/sections/codeswitch/2019/09/01/755629721/for-trans-women-silicone-pumping-can-be-a-blessing-and-a-curse. Accessed October 4, 2022.
4. Braley S. The status of injectable silicone fluid for soft tissue augmentation. Plast Reconstr Surg 1971;47(4):343–4.
5. Sergi FD, Wilson EC. Filler use among trans women: correlates of feminizing subcutaneous injections and their health consequences. Transgend Health 2021;6(2):82–90.
6. James SE, Herman JL, Rankin S, et al. Executive summary of the report of the 2015 U.S. Transgender survey. Washington, DC: National Center for Transgender Equality; 2016.
7. Coleman E, Radix AE, Bouman WP, et al. Standards of care for the health of transgender and gender diverse people, version 8. International Journal of Transgender Health 2022;23(Suppl 1):S1–259.
8. American Society of Plastic Surgeons. 2020 Plastic Surgery Statistics. Available at: https://www.plasticsurgery.org/documents/News/Statistics/2020/plastic-surgery-statistics-full-report-2020.pdf. Accessed October 2, 2022.
9. Goel A, Rai K. Male lip filler—Aesthetic enhancement is not just limited to females: a case report. J Cosmet Dermatol 2021;20:3173–6.
10. Ousterhout DK. Feminization of the forehead: contour changing to improve female aesthetics. Plast Reconstr Surg 1987;79(5):701–13.
11. Spiegel JH. Facial determinants of female gender and feminizing forehead cranioplasty. Laryngoscope 2011;121:250–61.
12. Viscomi B. From anatomical modifications to skin quality: case series of botulinum toxin and facial fillers for facial feminization in transgender women. Clin Cosmet Invest Dermatol 2022;15:1333–45.
13. Carruthers J, Carruthers A. Three-dimensional forehead reflation. Dermatol Surg 2015;41(Suppl 1):S321–4.
14. Tsukahara K, Hotta M, Osanai O, et al. Gender-dependent differences in degree of facial wrinkles. Skin Res Technol 2013;19:e65–71.
15. Bloom JD, Green JB, Bowe W, et al. Cosmetic use of abobotulinumtoxinA in men: considerations regarding anatomical differences and product characteristics. J Drugs Dermatol 2016;15(9):1056–62.
16. Flynn TC. Botox in men. Dermatol Ther 2007;20(6):407–13.
17. Carruthers A, Carruthers J. Prospective, double-blind, randomized, parllel-group, dose-ranging study of botulinum toxin type A in men with glabellar rhytids. Dermatol Surg 2005;31:1297–303.
18. de Maio M, Swift A, Signorini M, et al. Aesthetic Leaders in Facial Aesthetics Consensus C. Facial assessment and injection guide for botulinum toxin and injectable hyaluronic acid fillers: focus on the upper face. Plast Reconstr Surg 2017;140(2):265e–76e.
19. Moradi A, Shirazi A, Perez V. A guide to temporal fossa augmentation with small gel particle hyaluronic acid dermal filler. J Drugs Dermatol 2011;10(6):673–6.
20. Breithaupt AD, Jones DH, Braz A, et al. Anatomical basis for safe and effective volumization of the temple. Dermatol Surg 2015;41(Suppl 1):S278–83.
21. de Boulle K, Furuyama N, Heydenrych I, et al. Considerations for the use of minimally invasive aesthetic procedures for facial remodeling in transgender individuals. Clin Cosmet Invest Dermatol 2021;14:513–25.
22. Chronicle EP, Chan MY, Hawkings C, et al. You can tell by the nose—judging sex from an isolated facial feature. Perception 1995;24:969–73.
23. Flynn TC, Carruthers JA, Carruthers JA. Botulinum-A toxin treatment of the lower eyelid improves infraorbital rhytides and widens the eye. Dermatol Surg 2001;27:703–8.
24. Carruthers J, Rzany B, Sattler G, et al. Anatomic guidelines for augmentation of the cheek and infraorbital hollow. Dermatol Surg 2012;38:1223–33.
25. Thayer ZM, Dobson SD. Sexual dimorphism in chin shape: implications for adaptive hypotheses. Am J Phys Anthropol 2010;143:417–25.
26. Kundu N, Kothari R, Shah N, et al. Efficacy of botulinum toxin in masseter muscle hypertrophy for lower

face contouring. J Cosmet Dermatol 2022;21: 1849–56.

27. Braz A, Humphrey S, Weinkle S, et al. Lower face: clinical anatomy and regional approaches with injectable fillers. Plast Reconstr Surg 2015;136(5S):235S–57S.

28. Harview CL, Tan KW, Dhinsa HK, et al. The neurotoxin "Lip Flip": a case series and discussion. J Cosmet Dermatol 2021;20:3716–8.

29. Ginsberg BA. Dermatologic care of the transgender patient. Int J Womens Dermatol 2017;3:65–7.

30. Haedersdal M and Gøtzsche PC. Laser and photo-epilation for unwanted hair growth, *Cochrane Database Syst Rev*, (4), 2006, CD004684. Available at: https://www.cochranelibrary.com/cdsr/doi/10.1002/14651858.CD004684.pub2/full. Accessed October 5, 2022.

Feminization Rhinoplasty

A.J. Flaherty, MD[a],*, Ari M. Stone, MD[b], Jeffrey C. Teixeira, MD, MBA[c], Michael J. Nuara, MD[a,d]

KEYWORDS

- Rhinoplasty • Transgender • Facial feminization surgery • Gender affirmation
- Gender-affirming surgery • Gender-affirming facial surgery

KEY POINTS

- Transgender, nonbinary, and other gender-diverse people comprise a significant and growing proportion of the population. Gender-affirming care, an important tool for decreasing dysphoria and improving psychosocial function, consists of a wide variety of interventions developed to help align the features of an individual's assigned sex with their gender identity.
- A number of common rhinoplasty techniques can be used during feminization rhinoplasty to achieve common goals of dorsal reduction and symmetry, tip refinement and rotation, and decreasing alar width and flare. Although some feminization rhinoplasty can be managed quite simply, revision cases are best performed by a surgeon who is highly experienced in revision rhinoplasty.
- Feminization rhinoplasty often requires significant dorsal width reduction and/or deprojection, making certain complications more likely. Awareness of these risks and identification of their causes allows surgeons to prevent undesirable outcomes.

INTRODUCTION

Gender dysphoria, the psychological distress resulting from dissonance between an individual's gender and sex assigned at birth, causes significant functional impairment across multiple domains. Gender-affirming care (GAC) aims to relieve symptoms of dysphoria and improve quality of life.[1] Gender-affirming facial surgery (GAFS), an increasingly included part of gender affirmation, can involve a wide variety of procedures to feminize or masculinize the face.[2] During the past several years, facial feminization surgery (FFS) has emerged as an integral component of GAC for many trans women and transfeminine nonbinary individuals. As the central structure of the face, the nose plays a considerable role in patient and public perceptions of femininity and attractiveness. It is no surprise that rhinoplasty ranks among the most popular procedures within FFS, surpassed only by—and often performed in conjunction with—forehead and orbital contouring.[3]

HISTORY

Western medicine, as an extension of Western civilization, has historically established the experiences of heterosexual, cisgender, white men as the norm.[4] Analogous to the colonial invention of race as a concept,[5] Western imperialism created a gender binary that excludes the experiences of countless people who have long existed outside this dichotomy.[6] Examples of such "third gender" identities include the Hijra of India and Bangladesh, Fa'afafine of Samoa, two-spirit of precolonial North America, Māhū of Hawai'i and Tahiti, Xanith of Oman, Travesti of Brazil, and

[a] Facial Plastic & Reconstructive Surgery, Division of Otolaryngology - Head & Neck Surgery, Virginia Mason Medical Center, 1100 9th Avenue, Seattle, WA 98101, USA; [b] Department of Otolaryngology - Head and Neck Surgery, Southern Illinois University, 720 North Bond Street, Springfield, IL 62702, USA; [c] Uniformed Services University of the Health Science, 4301 Jones Bridge Road, Bethesda, MD 20814, USA; [d] University of Washington Department of Otolaryngology
* Corresponding author.
E-mail address: AJ.Flaherty@vmmc.org

Facial Plast Surg Clin N Am 31 (2023) 407–417
https://doi.org/10.1016/j.fsc.2023.04.005

Bissu and Waria of Indonesia.[7] Meanwhile, newer terms like "transgender" and "nonbinary," along with separate definitions for the social constructs of sex and gender, have developed in an effort to understand the existence of people who exist outside the gender binary.

BACKGROUND
Growing Awareness of Gender Diversity

A recent survey found that 5.1% of US adults under 30 years old identify as transgender or nonbinary.[8] Documented increases in the percentage of transgender and gender-diverse (TGD) people are anticipated to continue as societal shifts toward integration and appreciation of diversity encourage individuals to live openly as their true selves and as data collection methods improve.[9] Despite these strides in cultural inclusion, TGD patients continue to report lack of provider knowledge as the single greatest barrier to gender-affirming health care.[10,11] It is evident that the medical community will have to keep (or, at times, catch) up to effectively address the needs of this growing patient population.

Expanding Access and Rising Demand for Gender-affirming Care

Coverage options for GAC, although not universal, are more numerous than ever before. Following the 2014 Department of Health and Human Services' determination that exclusion of transition-related services under Medicare defied current standards of care, over a dozen states prohibited exclusion by third-party payers.[12] As of this writing, 26 states and the District of Columbia explicitly cover GAC under Medicaid.[13] While rates of all gender-affirming surgical procedures have increased correspondingly during the last 8 years, FFS has witnessed explosive demand. For example, although the number of augmentation mammoplasties performed for gender dysphoria nearly doubled between 2013 and 2018, the frequency of FFS increased almost 16-fold.[3] This trend is particularly surprising given insurance barriers unique to facial surgeries, which are routinely still designated as "nonessential" or "cosmetic," compared with other types of gender-affirming surgical care.[14]

Out of many possible explanations for the surge in FFS, its profound impact on dysphoria and social functioning is most apparent. Gender dysphoria is a highly individualized phenomenon, with no two patients likely to experience the exact same set of triggers and psychosocial consequences. In some TGD individuals, dysphoria may be strictly physical, with distress provoked by certain anatomic features associated with their assigned sex. Others may have solely social dysphoria. These patients, although comfortable with their physical characteristics, experience distress from misperception of their gender cues and identity (ie, misgendering) by others. For most TGD patients seeking GAC, dysphoria encompasses the dual discomfort of both bodily self-perception and public misgendering. Categorizing strangers into a binary sex is a subconscious and highly efficient cognitive process acquired in early childhood.[15] Since human sexual dimorphism is relatively subtle compared with other animal species, this process of pattern recognition relies heavily on the angles and proportions of the face for clues. This may explain why transgender women report facial appearance and facial hair among the most significant sources of dysphoria.[16]

Outcomes and Importance of Facial Feminization Surgery

Although feminizing hormone therapy can alter facial soft tissues by softening the skin and redistributing subcutaneous fat, it cannot change the underlying bony structure and proportions of the facial skeleton. FFS is a well-established treatment of gender dysphoria in transfeminine individuals with high rates of patient satisfaction.[14,17–19] Multiple studies have demonstrated significant postoperative reductions in anxiety, depression, and social isolation.[20,21] Of course, for many patients, the success of FFS is measured not only by their own satisfaction but by changes in public perception and treatment. In a recent survey, hundreds of participants were shown photos of cisgender men, cisgender women, and transgender women before and after FFS, then asked to categorize each face into a binary sex. Although about 1% of cisgender men and women were misgendered, almost half of transgender women were incorrectly identified as male in their preoperative photos despite make-up, feminine hairstyles, and hormone therapy. Rates of misgendering dropped precipitously—to 5.7%—among the postoperative photos.[22] For some individuals, these changes in public gender perception post-FFS may extend far beyond easing dysphoria and reducing social friction. TGD persons are more than 4 times more likely to be the victims of violent crime.[23] Those perceived to be transgender women, and particularly those who are Black and/or Latinx, are disproportionately targeted.[24] In patients at high risk for violence, FFS may be essential to ensuring physical safety.

Goals of Feminization Rhinoplasty

A wide range of procedures falls under FFS with a unifying goal to transform undesired masculine characteristics into more traditionally feminine ones. As the central structure of the midface, the nose occupies an important position in the perception of gender and overall attractiveness. Cephalometric studies have shown male noses to be, on average, larger and more angular, with either a straight profile or a dorsal hump. The masculine nasofrontal angle is smaller, owing to a more accentuated glabellar prominence. The nasolabial angle is also more acute in men (90°–95°) than in women (95°–105°), corresponding to less tip rotation and minimal to no supratip break.[12,18,22,25–28] The general goals of feminization rhinoplasty, then, are to reduce the overall size of the nose and nasal dorsum, refine and rotate the nasal tip, and accentuate the supratip break.[18,27] In the context of FFS, rhinoplasty is rarely performed as an isolated procedure. Combination with fronto-orbital reduction and/or lip lift enables the surgeon to increase the patient's nasofrontal and nasolabial angles, respectively. To achieve optimal results, feminization rhinoplasty may require more tissue reduction than a cosmetic rhinoplasty in a cisgender female patient.[29] This fact must be weighed against the risk of nasal valve collapse and loss of tip support; cartilage grafts should be used judiciously to avoid these sequelae.[18,26–28]

It should be noted that while cephalometric data can provide general guidelines, individual preferences and goals for embodying their gender may vary. Feminine beauty is not an indelible and singular ideal but a mutable concept across time and culture. Goals for female rhinoplasty were originally established through the lens of Eurocentric beauty standards. Because it relates to the concept of "ideal" nasal appearance, we witness cultural divergence and changing trends over time as we challenge the historical lens of Western social norms. What was once considered the "ideal" nose was driven by the perception of White (generally male) surgeons describing the White female nose. Even today, reports in the rhinoplasty literature refer to "ethnic rhinoplasty"[30] or "male rhinoplasty" to delineate this deviation from the historic gold standard. In the upcoming decades, we expect to see shifts in "ideal" nasal characteristicsbased on changing perspectives of gender norms. The past 20 years have witnessed an emergence of literature regarding the unique considerations for patients of color seeking rhinoplasty; however, there is still limited research specifically addressing non-White feminization rhinoplasty. Additionally, there is a dearth of information about the experiences of nonbinary people seeking rhinoplasty or gender affirming surgery in general. It is notable that about half of TGD youth and young adults currently identify as nonbinary.[8] As this population ages, surgical practice may evolve accordingly.

DISCUSSION
Patient Assessment and Counseling

Our approach to creating a welcoming, respectful, and gender-affirming environment for TGD patients starts with making a good first impression. The wording on a practice website or social media post, interactions between patients and call centers/front desk staff, and the design of waiting areas are intentionally built with inclusivity in mind. We engage in ongoing efforts to improve staff education, awareness, and sensitivity regarding the experiences of TGD individuals. All staff members are encouraged to wear badges identifying their own pronouns, to avoid assuming the gender and pronouns of others, and to ask politely when they are unsure. Intake forms specifically request chosen names, pronouns, and gender identity. For insurance purposes, legal names must be maintained in the electronic medical record (EMR) but chosen names are also documented and updated in the EMR as soon as they are available, even if not legally changed.

We begin each visit by confirming the patient's correct name and pronouns and their desire to discuss GAFS. Next, we elicit their specific postoperative goals. Many of our TGD patients identify strongly on the gender binary and wish to appear as feminine or as masculine as possible. Our practice has a growing cohort of patients who identify as nonbinary. Among this group, many still wish to appear maximally feminine or masculine, whereas others desire to have a more androgynous appearance, or perhaps only to address a specific facial characteristic that causes dysphoria. We ask each patient to identify which of their facial characteristics contribute to dysphoria and/or misgendering, as well as specific familial features they may wish to preserve. We also discuss relevant ethnic or cultural considerations that can influence patient expectations. In addition to a full medical history, we ask for any history of facial or nasal trauma or surgery, allergic rhinitis, and symptoms of functional nasal obstruction. Each patient completes Nasal Obstruction and Septoplasty Effectiveness (NOSE)[31] and Standardized Cosmesis and Health Nasal Outcomes Survey (SCHNOS)[32] forms to establish their baseline and track postoperative results.

Once we have developed a rapport with our patients and obtained the necessary history and physical examination, we discuss options for treatment. After emphasizing that not every patient needs or wants every intervention, we describe the options for GAFS available through our practice as well as some procedures (eg, hair transplantation) that are available via referral. We then narrow our focus to the patient's specific features that contribute to dysphoria, misgendering, and/or a facial appearance that does not align with their gender identity. Our surgical plan is thus individualized for each patient based on shared decision-making. If a patient desires gender-affirming rhinoplasty, we methodologically examine and formulate a plan for each aesthetic nasal characteristic. This involves measuring nasion depth; assessing dorsal projection and symmetry; palpating the width of the nasal bones; and noting tip shape, support, rotation, and projection. Factors contributing to nasal function are also documented, including dynamic collapse, septal position, turbinate size, the internal and external valves, and mucosal health.

Timing of the Rhinoplasty

Timing must be considered because it relates to both the patient's stage of transition as well as the sequence of other gender-affirming facial procedures. There are no set guidelines as to when FFS should be performed. For patients planning to begin feminizing hormone therapy, we encourage them to prioritize doing so before FFS; the associated changes in hairline position, hair density, skin texture, and facial fat distribution after 1 to 2 years of consistent hormone replacement can influence surgical planning and recovery. However, assuming a patient is otherwise medically optimized, the decision on when to proceed with facial surgery is largely a matter of personal preference. We therefore do not require hormone therapy before GAFS.

As with any rhinoplasty, there are several considerations regarding patient age at the time of surgery. For example, it is rarely appropriate to consider non-functional rhinoplasty in a prepubescent child. Hormonal influences on facial development and growth far outstrip any surgical manipulations that can be made and long-term results are minimally predictable. In adolescents, the decision about when to proceed with rhinoplasty requires careful discussion. For example, definitive feminizing rhinoplasty may be considered in a teenage patient on long-term hormone therapy, for whom the influences of endogenous testosterone are minimized. The latest update to

Standards of Care for the Health of Transgender and Gender Diverse People (SOC-8) recommends that adolescents have "at least 12 months of gender-affirming hormone therapy or longer, if required, to achieve the desired surgical result for gender-affirming procedures, including… facial surgery as part of gender-affirming treatment unless hormone therapy is either not desired or is medically contraindicated."[9] The rationale for this guideline mirrors our own recommendations for preoperative hormone therapy.

Factors that may influence the decision to proceed with isolated rhinoplasty before other FFS procedures may include the patient's relative needs and desires, the extent of surgery required to reach the desired outcome, and the presence of nasal obstruction or deformity that would otherwise be considered an indication for surgery at this age. For instance, in a nonbinary adolescent with notable nasal incongruence deformity, isolated rhinoplasty may be the least invasive pathway to gender affirmation and dysphoria relief at an age before significant psychosocial damage has occurred. Similarly, if the degree of surgery required to meet the patient's overall needs is significant and there is coexisting congenital or traumatic nasal deformity, a staged procedure may be the best option to avoid surgeon fatigue and achieve ideal results. Finally, if a functional rhinoplasty is indicated to correct severe nasal obstruction, it may be appropriate to include gender affirmation goals in the surgical plan even for younger patients, in order to avoid the need for a future revision rhinoplasty. This is particularly true in the case of severe traumatic deformity, congenital nasal deformity, or as part of a comprehensive management plan to address obstructive sleep apnea. These decisions generally come about as part of a multidisciplinary consensus.

Timing of rhinoplasty within a sequence of comprehensive GAFS is also important. A variety of approaches to FFS have been described, including top-down, bottom-up, and inside-out sequencing. In a top-down approach, the forehead and hairline are addressed before the mandible and nose. Bottom-up approaches reverse this order. The authors prefer an inside-out approach, with the larynx addressed first, followed by the mandible through the oral cavity, then the forehead and orbits through a scalp/hairline incision. After fronto-orbital reduction, one surgeon begins rhinoplasty while other members of the team complete the scalp/hairline closure. The central location of the nose makes it difficult to avoid when retracting or manipulating the face during other procedures. We therefore recommend addressing the nose after working in the oral cavity, and after the forehead skin has been redraped, to avoid incidental distortion with retraction. This approach additionally allows for superior access to the nasion and nasal bones during fronto-orbital contouring, enabling efficient overlap of surgical tasks.

RHINOPLASTY TECHNIQUES

A number of common rhinoplasty techniques can be used during feminization rhinoplasty to achieve common goals of dorsal reduction and symmetry, tip refinement and rotation, and decreasing alar width and flare. Depending on individual patient anatomy and desired outcomes, either open or endonasal approaches may be used. In the patient with relatively good symmetry who desires a simple reduction rhinoplasty, an endonasal approach is usually recommended. In most cases, a structural component resection technique is preferred over dorsal preservation, as the latter is difficult via endonasal exposure and rarely adequate to address the testosterone-induced width of the keystone region. Bilateral medial and lateral marginal incisions afford broad exposure of the lower lateral cartilages (LLCs), upper lateral cartilages (ULCs), and bony dorsum. Intercartilaginous or transcartilaginous incisions can often be avoided because the excess skin envelope resulting from dorsal reduction allows for similar exposure to open techniques through the marginal incisions alone. However, such incisions may be added to aid in tip delivery, especially if significant tip work is needed.

The open approach provides the broadest exposure yet adds to surgical time and postoperative edema. Although comprehensive FFS (e.g., hairline advancement, fronto-orbital reduction/cranioplasty, rhinoplasty, malar augmentation, lip lift/augmentation, genioplasty and mandibular reduction, submental liposuction, laryngeal chondroplasty) can be performed in a single operation, surgical times frequently exceed 8 hours. The reality of surgeon fatigue must be considered and efforts made to reduce surgical time without compromising results. Regardless, if there is a significant dorsal or caudal deviation, an open approach is still preferred.

Reduction can be accomplished by sharply opening the middle vault followed by serial excision of the dorsal septum (and ULCs, if needed). The bony dorsum can be reduced with a rasp, osteotome, or powered instrumentation, often resulting in a bilateral medial osteotomy. The authors typically then reconstruct the middle vault with spreader grafts, autospreader flaps, or simply by suturing the ULCs to the new dorsal septum,

before proceeding with lateral osteotomies and tip refinement. However, this sequencing depends on the surgeon's individual skills and preferences and generally does not differ significantly from how the operation may unfold when performed for other indications.

Addressing the bony vault is necessary to establish the classical hourglass appearance of the brow-tip aesthetic lines which are wider at the glabella, narrow through the midvault, and then wider again at the tip. When feminizing rhinoplasty is performed as a component of comprehensive FFS, a transverse osteotomy is made during fronto-orbital contouring, given the superior access to the nasion and cephalad aspect of the nasal bones compared to other traditional rhinoplasty approaches (**Fig. 1**). Subsequently, any significant nasal bone asymmetry can be addressed with an intermediate osteotomy.[33]

The "x-point," or the nasal base at the nasomaxillary junction, should be roughly two-thirds of the alar base. Lateral osteotomies are typically needed to narrow the bony vault, improve dorsal aesthetic lines, and close any open roof deformity resulting from dorsal reduction. However, although most traditional rhinoplasty techniques use the "high-low-high" pathway to preserve the x-point width and lateral suspensory ligament attachments,[34] the senior author often performs a more lateral osteotomy for feminization rhinoplasty. Doing so reduces the position of the x-point and medializes the overly wide nasal pyramid. This maneuver is performed with great care and in conjunction with any other functional procedures as necessary with the goal of narrowing the nasal vault while avoiding functional compromise. Alternatively, spreader grafting can be used after

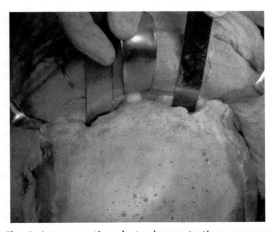

Fig. 1. Intraoperative photo demonstrating exposure for fronto-orbital contouring/cranioplasty with access to the radix and cephalad aspect of the nasal bones.

significant dorsal reduction to establish appropriate and balanced brow-tip aesthetic lines without narrowing the nasal base.

Tip refinement is typically required and may include both cephalic adjustments and/or a combination of tip sutures or continuous strip techniques to adjust the LLCs. A combination of multiple techniques can be used to simultaneously deproject the tip while increasing rotation; however, structural grafting is rarely necessary in the absence of additional indications to treat functional obstruction. Dividing the lateral crus 3 to 4 mm cephalic and parallel to the tip defining point, then advancing the lateral segment in underlay fashion to the medial segment, can control rotation and deprojection while also contributing to a supratip break. Additional rotation can be attained as needed by trimming the lateral segment before the underlay advancement, and enhanced with intradomal sutures. Similarly, if there is a greater need for deprojection, the medial crura can be trimmed at the infratip lobule. Tensioning sutures or cephalic turnover flaps are added as needed to adjust lateral crural convexity.[35] We agree with previous reports that tongue and groove positioning of the medial crura is a powerful maneuver to set final tip position and we incorporate this into most feminization rhinoplasties.[36] Furthermore, tongue and groove positioning can aid with sustaining tip position, especially after significant tip manipulation such as with vertical dome division.[37]

Although most feminization rhinoplasty requires significant reduction, variable anatomy can necessitate alternative approaches. Anatomic nasal classifications are generally more useful than those based on concepts of race or ethnicity.[30] The leptorrhine patient is more likely to benefit from the reduction of an overprojected dorsum and tip, whereas a platyrrhine nose may be adequately feminized by increasing tip projection and adjusting nostril shape. Meanwhile, the in-between mesorrhine patient might require a combination of dorsal reduction with an increased tip rotation and projection (**Fig. 2**). Leptorrhine and mesorrhine noses have variable skin thickness, are more prone to tip ptosis, and have alar positioning which often approximates intercanthal distance (**Fig. 3**). Platyrrhine noses tend to have thicker skin and weaker cartilage with flattened, flared, and horizontally shaped nostrils which result in more a wide-set position of the alar crease.

The alar base can serve as a set point for other rhinoplasty measurements, such as nasal bone width, and should be addressed if excessively wide. It is important to differentiate between a wide alar base (ie, the distance between each alar crease) versus alar flaring. Excessive alar flaring refers to the convexity of the alar edge extending more than 2 mm lateral to the alar crease. A wide alar base can be narrowed using nostril sill reduction in which a 1 to 4 mm wedge of tissue is removed. On the other hand, alar flaring can be addressed with alar wedge excision, in which an elliptical excision is placed in the alar crease toreduce the vertical length of the alar lobule. These procedures may be combined in patients who have both a wide alar base and alar flaring. Nostril orientation and symmetry can be improved by adjusting the amount of reduction performed on each side.[38] It is also important to note that some deprojection maneuvers can result in alar flaring that requires adjustment. We often perform lip lift in conjunction with feminizing rhinoplasty as a part of comprehensive FFS. Placing the lip lift incision in the alar crease and nasal sill hides the scar within these natural creases and allows for moderate narrowing of the alar base when the nasal sill incisions are planned appropriately. However, attempting to reduce the sill more than 2 mm on each side using the lip lift incision alone has been noted to distort the alar margin. In these cases, complete release of the alar attachment is required to avoid distortion.

Functional Nasal Considerations

As in cosmetic rhinoplasty, the surgeon must work to achieve aesthetic outcomes without compromising function. We identify and document functional concerns during our initial patient assessments, use NOSE and SCHNOS forms to track postoperative outcomes, and discuss with each patient how feminization rhinoplasty often requires maneuvers that can compromise nasal function. We advocate for balancing the constantly evolving push for smaller and more feminine noses with the functionality of nasal breathing. Therefore, if septal deviation is found on examination, even in the absence of preoperative symptoms or dorsal deviation, we strongly recommend concomitant septoplasty to prevent functional nasal obstruction that would be anticipated to result from reduction rhinoplasty alone.

Septoplasty can be approached through the same combination of endonasal incisions described above or by adding a transfixion incision. We recommend performing dorsal reduction before septoplasty and tip work to allow for an expanded exposure.This aids other aspects of the procedure when performed endonasally and will ensure maintenance of an adequate dorsal strut . In individuals who have had previous septoplasty, dorsal reduction may result in an

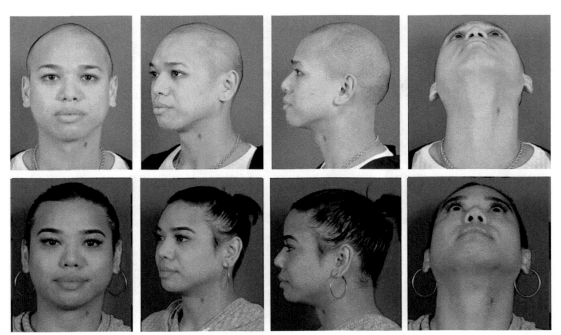

Fig. 2. A 30-year-old transgender Filipina woman. Top row: characteristics of a mesorrhine nose, featuring mild dorsal prominence, wide-set nasal bones caudally, and wide, underrotated, deprojected tip. Bottom row: 7 weeks after open reduction rhinoplasty with minimal rasping of mild dorsal prominence, caudal septal extension graft with tongue-in-groove suture and 2 interdomal sutures (used to increase tip rotation and projection), medial and lateral (high-low-high) osteotomies (used to narrow the caudal aspect of the nasal bones), and functional septoplasty. Additional procedures included laryngeal chondroplasty, submental liposuction, reduction genioplasty and mandibular osteoplasty, mandibular angle reduction with masseter muscle resection, hairline advancement, forehead reduction with frontal sinus setback, bilateral browlift, and autologous fat grafting to the malar regions.

inadequate dorsal strut; Tand thus, the surgeon must be prepared to reconstruct the "L" strut, which may require autologous cartilage grafting or extracorporeal techniques. Although some reduction feminization rhinoplasty can be managed quite simply, revision cases are best performed by a surgeon who is highly experienced in revision rhinoplasty.

Consideration of Other Feminizing Facial Procedures

Typical exposure for fronto-orbital reduction/cranioplasty includes subperiosteal dissection onto the nasal root to expose the entire glabella and nasofrontal suture line. As mentioned previously, this allows access to the cephalad aspect of the nasal dorsum and sidewalls (see **Fig. 1**). Such radix exposure is equivalent in extent and in some ways superior in symmetry (allowing a view of anatomy from midline without having to lean over or turn the head of the patient) compared with operating from either side of the patient. When combining feminizing cranioplasty and rhinoplasty

in a single operation, the authors prefer to complete as much of the superior rhinoplasty as possible via cranioplasty exposure. Then, after redraping the forehead skin, the remaining aspects of the rhinoplasty can be completed from below, maintaining the position of the cranioplasty. This applies to both structural and dorsal preservation rhinoplasty approaches. For the same reason, we typically avoid placing any reconstructive hardware used for the cranioplasty onto the nasal root. The final step of the cranioplasty involves application of bone pâté over the frontal sinus osteotomy sites. This is best applied after completing the transverse nasal osteotomy and cephalad dorsal reduction to avoid disruption of the bone pâté before scalp closure.

The authors perform lip lift after rhinoplasty as one of the last steps of comprehensive FFS, followed only by autologous fat grafting to the malar regions and lips, if necessary. The senior author has modified the traditional bullhorn shape to use a geometric broken line incision placed in the nasal sill instead of curved lines inferior to the sill, and extends the curved lateral incisions further into

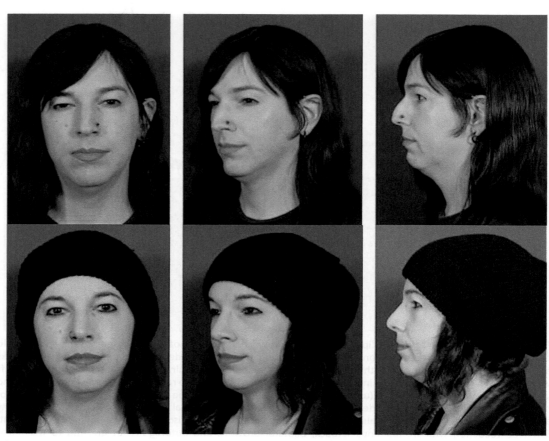

Fig. 3. A 41-year-old transgender woman. Top row: characteristics of a leptorrhine nose, featuring overprojected dorsum and long LLCs with tip ptosis. Bottom row: 3 months after open reduction rhinoplasty with dorsal reduction using the Rubin osteotome and a rasp (resulting in medial osteotomies), lateral osteotomies, autospreader flaps, lateral crural steal (to reposition the tip defining point and increase rotation and projection), and functional septoplasty. She additionally underwent a transblepharoplasty approach to frontal bar contouring and browpexy.

the alar crease (**Figs. 4** and **5**). As previously noted, placing the lip lift incision in the nasal sill hides the scar within the nose and allows for moderate narrowing of the alar base when the nasal sill incisions are planned appropriately. Extending the lateral aspects of the incision superiorly into the alar crease results in a greater lateral lifting effect on the upper lip. We agree with previous reports regarding the safety of performing lip lift after open rhinoplasty and do so regularly without complications.[39] One of the more significant risks of lip lift is scar widening or hypertrophy resulting in an obvious incision. We mitigate this risk bycombining the geometric incision with the use of careful buried dermal sutures to minimize tension on the closure without undermining, which would negate the procedure's lifting effect. Lip lift can be performed at the same time as alar flare reduction with wedge excision, yet careful suturing is required to set the new alar base in the alar crease

given the shared position of the lip lift incision within the alar crease. The tension of the lip lift in the alar crease is directed inferolaterally, whereas the tension of the wedge excision is directed

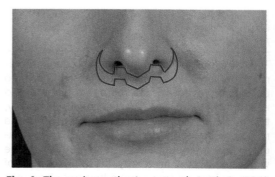

Fig. 4. The senior author's approach to designing a geometric broken line lip lift incision placed in the nasal sill, with curved lateral incisions extending into the alar crease.

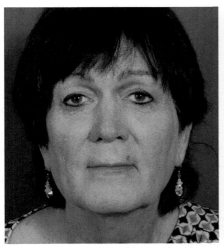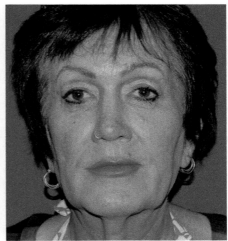

Fig. 5. A 60-year-old transgender woman, before (*left*) and 2 months after in-office lip lift (*right*) while awaiting insurance authorization for other FFS procedures.

superomedially. Carefully placed sutures can adequately counter these opposing forces, preventing scar widening, nostril asymmetry, and lip lift asymmetry.

Complications

Complications associated with feminizing rhinoplasty are similar to those seen in rhinoplasty performed for cosmetic and functional indications, including infection, bleeding, septal perforation, cartilage warping or resorption, poor cosmetic outcomes, and need for revision surgery. However, certain complications may develop more commonly in feminizing rhinoplasty due to the nature of the operation. Testosterone effects on the nose during puberty often result in a large dorsal hump and widened midvault, which must be reduced to achieve a feminine-appearing nose. Significant dorsal hump reduction can result in open roof deformity; this should be prevented by closing osteotomies and/or using spreader grafts. Reducing a large nose by narrowing the midvault and nasal bone width can compromise the cross-sectional area of the nasal cavity and contribute to functional nasal obstruction. While reduction can also cause internal nasal valve collapse, appropriate middle vault reconstruction can prevent compromising nasal breathing. Disrupting the ULCs from their connection to the caudal end of the nasal bones leads to inverted-V deformity if this relationship is not reestablished. During endonasal approaches, the senior author often avoids elevating the mucoperichondrium along the dorsal septum under the ULCs. Aesthetic goals must be balanced with functional outcomes and other anatomic factors that contribute to obstruction (eg, septal deviation,

inferior turbinate hypertrophy) should be identified and treated. Finally, alterations in nostril shape can result from the significant deprojection that feminization rhinoplasty often requires but can be ameliorated using a variety of methods as described above.

SUMMARY

As the population of TGD patients continues to grow, we anticipate an increasing demand for gender-affirming surgical care, including GAFS, over the coming decades. Among the most popular FFS procedures, feminization rhinoplasty uses a variety of established techniques to achieve common goals of dorsal reduction and symmetry, tip refinement and rotation, and decreasing alar width and flare. It is often performed in combination with other feminizing facial procedures, allowing for adjustment of the nasofrontal angle that cannot be attained by rhinoplasty alone. The nature of the operation makes certain complications more likely but awareness of these risks and identification of their causes allows for prevention. Although the individual surgeon's skills and preferences may guide their approach to feminizing rhinoplasty, revision cases are best performed by a surgeon who is highly experienced in revision rhinoplasty.

CLINICS CARE POINTS

- More than 5% of US adults aged younger than 30 years identify as transgender or nonbinary.

- FFS is a well-established treatment of facial gender dysphoria in transfeminine individuals with high rates of patient satisfaction and clinically significant reductions in anxiety, depression, and social isolation.
- Feminization rhinoplasty is among the top 3 procedures performed within FFS. It is frequently combined with fronto-orbital reduction and/or lip lift.
- A number of common rhinoplasty techniques can be used during feminization rhinoplasty to achieve common goals of dorsal reduction and symmetry, tip refinement and rotation, and decreasing alar width and flare.
- Complications associated with reduction techniques may be more likely in feminization rhinoplasty but can be anticipated and prevented.

DISCLOSURE

The authors have no conflicts of interest or financial relationships to report.

REFERENCES

1. Reisner SL, Radix A, Deutsch MB. Integrated and Gender-Affirming Transgender Clinical Care and Research. J Acquir Immune Defic Syndr 2016; 72(Suppl 3):S235–42.
2. Deschamps-Braly. Facial Gender Confirmation Surgery: Facial Feminization Surgery and Facial Masculinization Surgery. Clin Plast Surg 2018;45(3): 323–31.
3. Chaya BF, Berman ZP, Boczar D, et al. Current Trends in Facial Feminization Surgery: An Assessment of Safety and Style. J Craniofac Surg 2021; 32(7):2366–9.
4. Silvano G. A brief history of Western medicine. Journal of Traditional Chinese Medical Sciences 2021; 8(Supplement 1):S10–6.
5. Roediger DR. Historical Foundations of Race. In: Smithsonian National Museum of African American history & culture. Available at: https://nmaahc.si. edu/learn/talking-about-race/topics/historical-foundations-race. Accessed October 5, 2022.
6. Urquhart I. Exploring the history of gender expression. In: Link, University of California Office of the President. 2019. Available at: https://link.ucop.edu/ 2019/10/14/exploring-the-history-of-gender-expression/. Accessed October 5, 2022.
7. Nanda S. Gender Diversity. In: Turner BS, editor. The Wiley-Blackwell encyclopedia of social theory. John Wiley & Sons, Ltd.; 2017. p. 1–3.
8. Brown A. About 5% of young adults in the U.S. say their gender is different from their sex assigned at birth. In:Pew Research Center, Pew Research Center. Available at: https://www.pewresearch.org/ fact-tank/2022/06/07/about-5-of-young-adults-in-the-u-s-say-their-gender-is-different-from-their-sex-assigned-at-birth/. Accessed October 5, 2022.
9. Coleman E, Radix AE, Bouman WP, et al. Standards of Care for the Health of Transgender and Gender Diverse People, Version 8. Int J Transgend Health 2022;23(Suppl 1):S1–259.
10. Winter S, Diamond M, Green J, et al. Transgender people: health at the margins of society. Lancet 2016;388(10042):390–400.
11. Safer JD, Tangpricha V. Care of the Transgender Patient. Ann Intern Med 2019;171(1):ITC1.
12. Safa B, Lin WC, Salim AM, et al. Current Concepts in Feminizing Gender Surgery. Plast Reconstr Surg 2019;143(5):1081e–91e.
13. Movement Advancement Project. Equality maps: healthcare laws and policies. Updated October 25, 2022. Available at: https://www.lgbtmap.org/ equality-maps/healthcare_laws_and_policies. Accessed October 26, 2022.
14. Caprini R, Oberoi M, Dejam D, et al. Effect of Gender-affirming Facial Feminization Surgery on Psychosocial Outcomes. Ann Surg 2022. https:// doi.org/10.1097/SLA.0000000000005472. Publish Ahead of Print.
15. Sykes JM, Dilger AE, Sinclair A. Surgical Facial Esthetics for Gender Affirmation. Dermatol Clin 2020; 38(2):261–8.
16. van de Grift TC, Cohen-Kettenis PT, Steensma TD, et al. Body Satisfaction and Physical Appearance in Gender Dysphoria. Arch Sex Behav 2016;45(3): 575–85.
17. Morrison S, Capitán-Cañadas F, Sánchez-Garcia A. et al. Prospective Quality-of-Life Outcomes after Facial Feminization Surgery: An International Multicenter Study. Plast Reconstr Surg 2020;145(6): 1499–509.
18. Bellinga R, Capitán L, Simon D, et al. Technical and Clinical Considerations for Facial Feminization Surgery With Rhinoplasty and Related Procedures. JAMA Facial Plast Surg 2017;19(3):175–81.
19. Weissler J, Chang B, Carney M, et al. Gender-Affirming Surgery in Persons with Gender Dysphoria. Plast Reconstr Surg 2018;141(3):388e–96e.
20. Esmonde N, Najafian A, Penkin A, et al. The Role of Facial Gender Confirmation Surgery in the Treatment of Gender Dysphoria. J Craniofac Surg 2019;30(5): 1387–92.
21. Ainsworth TA, Spiegel JH. Quality of life of individuals with and without facial feminization surgery or gender reassignment surgery. Qual Life Res 2010; 19(7):1019–24.
22. Fisher M, Lu SM, Chen K, et al. Facial Feminization Surgery Changes Perception of Patient Gender. Aesthetic Surg J 2020;40(7):703–9.

23. Williams Institute, UCLA School of Law. Transgender people over four times more likely than cisgender people to be victims of violent crime. March 23, 2021. Available at: https://williamsinstitute.law.ucla.edu/press/ncvs-trans-press-release.Accessed October 20, 2022.

24. Gyamerah A, Baguso G, Santiago-Rodriguez E, et al. Experiences and factors associated with transphobic hate crimes among transgender women in the San Francisco Bay Area: comparisons across race. BMC Publ Health 2021;21(1):1053.

25. Spiegel JH. Rhinoplasty as a Significant Component of Facial Feminization and Beautification. JAMA Facial Plast Surg 2017;19(3):181–2.

26. Becking AG, Tuinzing DB, Hage JJ, et al. Transgender feminization of the facial skeleton. Clin Plast Surg 2007;34(3):557–64.

27. Akhavan AA, Sandhu S, Ndem I, et al. A review of gender affirmation surgery: What we know, and what we need to know. Surgery 2021;170(1):336–40.

28. Nouraei SAR, Randhawa P, Andrews PJ, et al. The Role of Nasal Feminization Rhinoplasty in Male-to-Female Gender Reassignment. Arch Facial Plast Surg 2007;9(5):318–20.

29. Spiegel JH. Considerations in Feminization Rhinoplasty. Facial Plast Surg 2020;36(1):53–6.

30. Cobo R. Ethnic Rhinoplasty. Facial Plast Surg 2019;35(4):313–21.

31. Stewart MG, Witsell DL, Smith TL, et al. Development and validation of the Nasal Obstruction Symptom Evaluation (NOSE) Scale. Otolaryngol Head Neck Surg 2004;130(2):157–63.

32. Moubayed SP, Ioannidis JPA, Saltychev M, et al. The 10-Item Standardized Cosmesis and Health Nasal Outcomes Survey (SCHNOS) for Functional and Cosmetic Rhinoplasty. JAMA Facial Plast Surg 2018;20(1):37–42.

33. Ghanaatpisheh M, Sajjadian A, Daniel RK. Superior rhinoplasty outcomes with precise nasal osteotomy: an individualized approach for maintaining function and achieving aesthetic goals. Aesthet Surg J 2015;35(1):28–39.

34. Most SP, Murakami CS. A modern approach to nasal osteotomies. Facial Plast Surg Clin North Am 2005;13(1):85–92.

35. Murakami CS, Barrera JE, Most SP. Preserving structural integrity of the alar cartilage in aesthetic rhinoplasty using a cephalic turn-in flap. Arch Facial Plast Surg 2009;11(2):126–8.

36. Spataro EA, Most SP. Tongue-in-Groove Technique for Rhinoplasty: Technical Refinements and Considerations. Facial Plast Surg 2018;34(5):529–38.

37. Spataro EA, Most SP. Nuances of the Tongue-in-Groove Technique for Controlling Tip Projection and Rotation. JAMA Facial Plast Surg 2019;21(1):73–4.

38. Cerkes N. Alar Base Reduction: Nuances and Techniques. Clin Plast Surg 2022;49(1):161–78.

39. Insalaco L, Spiegel JH. Safety of Simultaneous Lip-Lift and Open Rhinoplasty. JAMA Facial Plast Surg 2017;19(2):160–1.

Gender Facial Affirmation Surgery; Techniques for Feminizing the Chin

Maggie Wanhe Wang, BA, Regina E. Rodman, MD*

KEYWORDS

- Feminization surgery • Facial feminization • Genioplasty • Sliding genioplasty
- Advancement genioplasty • Osseous genioplasty • Mandible reduction
- Facial feminization surgery

KEY POINTS

- Different variations of the osseous genioplasty can be used to feminize the chin and as a result, the overall appearance of a female transgender patient.
- The author describes 3 methods of genioplasty which change the projection, shape and width of the chin in different ways.
- The 3-piece genioplasty is often performed in combination with mandible reduction in a surgery known as V-line surgery
- Protection of the mental nerve and resuspension of the mentalis muscle are essential in order to avoid complications such as permanent lower lip numbness and ptosis respectively.

INTRODUCTION

Visibly prominent differences exist between the appearance of a typically male or female chin.[1] The male chin is generally broader and wider, has greater anterior projection than the female chin and is about 17% taller – traits that collectively contribute to a larger and more square appearance. The female chin, however, is typically more narrow, pointed, tapered, and shorter.[2] Because of its noted importance in gender identification, contouring of the chin is frequently an important aspect of facial feminization surgery. Lowering the height of the chin, reducing its width, or changing the degree of anterior projection by even a few millimeters can dramatically alter the perception of a female transgender patient.[3]

The options for chin augmentation include osseous genioplasty, a chin implant, or a combination of the 2. The most notable difference between the insertion of a chin implant and an osseous genioplasty is that with a chin implant, the appearance of the chin can only be altered via the addition of volume. For female transgender patients who desire a reduction in the size of their chin in addition to a change in shape, an osseous genioplasty is the only means of remodeling the chin in 3-dimensions.[4] Genioplasty can also be performed in conjunction with mandibular angle osteotomy or contouring – a set of procedures collectively termed V-line surgery (**Fig. 1**).[5] This is performed on patients with a significant lateral prominence on the back of the mandible, creating the appearance of a "square" jaw. Many female transgender patients feel that this contributes to their overall masculine appearance.

This article describes the procedure and efficacy of 3 types of osseous genioplasty performed by the senior author designed to contribute to a more feminine appearance. The first variation – termed the 1-piece genioplasty – is performed with recontouring through surface burring while

Face Forward Houston, 1900 North Loop W Suite 370, Houston, TX 77018, USA
* Corresponding author.
E-mail address: dr.rodman@faceforwardhouston.com

Facial Plast Surg Clin N Am 31 (2023) 419–431
https://doi.org/10.1016/j.fsc.2023.04.006
1064-7406/23/© 2023 Elsevier Inc. All rights reserved.

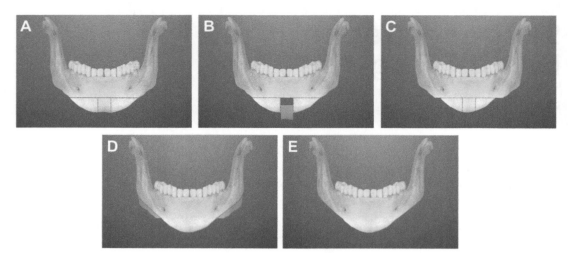

Fig. 1. (*A*) 3D model of the mandible with dotted denoting lines along which osteotomy is performed in a V-line surgery. (*B*) Red medial segment is removed from the free inferior portion of the mandible. (*C*) Lateral posterior wings of the mandible are removed. (*D*) Resulting V-shaped mandible. (*E*) Final result.

the latter 2 – termed the 2-piece genioplasty and 3-piece genioplasty – involve osteotomies that restructure the bone of the chin in all dimensions.

History

The osseous genioplasty was first described by Hofer in 1942[6] using an extraoral approach. Trauner and Obwegesser later improved this surgical procedure in 1957[7] such that it could be used to correct chin abnormalities such as microgenia. This adaptation allowed for chin augmentation in all 3 spatial planes via an intraoral approach. Later, in the 1980s, a notable improvement to prior wire fixation was introduced with the advent of plate and screw fixing.[8] The importance of using programs for digital imaging and planning in 2 and 3 dimensions has, in recent years, become increasingly emphasized in the preoperative planning of osseous genioplasties.[9–11]

Anatomy

The midline anterior projection of the mandible comprises the mental protuberance, commonly referred to as the chin. In addition to bone, the chin contains the premental fat pad, and a pair of muscles in the medial portion of the lower lip: the mentalis and depressor labii inferioris.

Muscles

The muscle most relevant to genioplasty is the mentalis muscle, as this muscle must be divided and repaired in the course of every genioplasty performed through an intraoral incision. The mentalis muscle originates from the mandibular incisive fossa before descending and inserting into the chin's dermis. In addition to elevating and protruding the lower lip, contraction of the mentalis muscle also causes the characteristic "orange peel" dimpling of the skin covering the chin. While genioplasty may improve mentalis strain, some patients will still require neuromodulators after surgery to reduce the dimpling of the chin. The mentalis muscle must be carefully resuspended and repaired in every case. Without resuspension, genioplasty patients are at risk of chin ptosis, or witch's chin.[12]

In addition to the mentalis, the depressor labii inferioris originates from the oblique line of the mandible in front of the mental foramen, passing upward and medially to insert into the skin of the lower lip, mucosa, and orbicularis oris fibers. Along with the suprahyoid muscle group (the anterior belly of digastric, mylohyoid, and geniohyoid), which attaches to the posterior aspect of the mandible, the depressor anguli oris (DAO), depressor labii inferioris (DLI), and genioglossus muscles also surround the osseous complex of the chin.

Nerves

The nerve most relevant to genioplasty is the mental nerve, as this must be avoided and protected during genioplasty. The mental nerve is the terminal branch of the inferior alveolar nerve. It transmits sensation from the mandibular incisor, the premolar teeth, the labial gingivae, as well as the skin that covers the chin and lower lip. The mental nerve exits the mandible through the mental foramen, which is situated bilaterally between the roots of the first and second premolar teeth at the level of the mentalis muscle origin. There, it divides

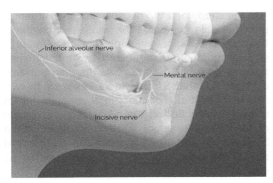

Fig. 2. Intramandibular course of the mental nerve dips about 5 mm below where the extramandibular course exits the mental foramen.

into 3 terminal branches beneath the DAO muscle. Notably, the intramandibular course of the nerve extends inferiorly about 5 mm below the foramen before extending superiorly and posteriorly through the body of the mandible (Fig. 2). This is important to note in surgical planning, as the osteotomy should be > 5 mm below the mental foramen to avoid cutting the nerve in its intraosseous course.[13]

Vasculature

Blood supply to the chin and lower lip is provided by both the mental artery branch of the inferior alveolar artery and the submental branch of the facial artery (Fig. 3). Once the inferior portion of the chin is separated from the mandible after the osteotomy, it does not receive any direct blood supply. The main source of blood supply is through the soft tissue attachment to the

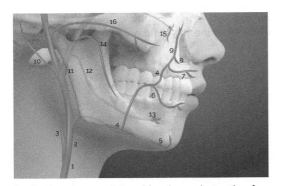

Fig. 3. Arteries providing blood supply to the face. 1 = common carotid, 2 = external carotid, 3 = internal carotid, 4 = facial, 5 = submental, 6 = inferior labial, 7 = superior labial, 8 = lateral Nasal, 9 = angular, 10 = posterior auricular, 11 = maxillary, 12 = inferior alveolar, 13 = mental, 14 = buccal, 15 = infraorbital, 16 = transverse facial.

periosteum. It is therefore essential to leave as much mucosa attached as possible.[14]

DISCUSSION
Evaluation

Preoperatively, a full history and physical are obtained from each patient. Patients are asked if they have had previous surgery to the face, previous orthodontics, or significant dental history. The physical exam should include Angle's classification of dental occlusion, oropharyngeal exam, tongue and floor of the mouth as well as the state of dentition. The genioplasty should not affect or change any of the above, but it is important to note and document any irregularities before surgery. Patients with multiple caries or dental decay should have these treated before considering any surgery to the mandible, as dental bacteria may seed the surgical field and create issues with healing.

In this practice, a CT scan is not required for genioplasty. A CT scan may be beneficial in revision cases, previous orthognathic surgery, or previous trauma. In these cases, a CT is used to assess the location of hardware, previous osteotomies, the integrity of the nerve foramen and canal, and any other factors that may complicate future surgery. If a CT scan is obtained for other surgical planning to be combined with the genioplasty, it is reviewed to assess asymmetry, the path of the mental nerve, and to rule out any abnormalities.

There is a rise in interest in virtual surgical planning with custom cutting guides and plates in recent years. The senior author does not use virtual surgical planning (VSP) for genioplasty due to the very high, and often unnecessary cost. While there may be benefits to using VSP at training institutions,[15] the VSP doubles or triples the cost of the operation, often making the surgery unaffordable for many patients. Without VSP, measurements and surgical decisions are performed intraoperatively. The senior author's observation has been that with experience, intraoperative decision-making is equally time-effective, equally safe, and more cost-effective.

In addition to standard consultation on the risks and benefits of the procedure, patients are counseled on the best type of procedure to suit their aesthetic goals. The decision regarding which technique to use depends on both the patient's anatomy and the patient's desired outcome. This practice has come to use the terms "1, 2, and 3-piece genioplasty" to differentiate the techniques.

One-piece Genioplasty

For patients with a prominent and pointed chin, excessive anterior projection, or a squared shape

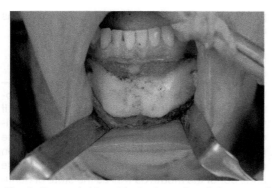

Fig. 4. Exposed chin with the integrity of the mental nerve preserved bilaterally.

and who would like a *round* appearance, the senior author advises what we call the 1-piece genioplasty. The 1-piece consists of surface burring only and no osteotomies are performed. The effect of this is a decrease in projection, often a decrease in vertical height, and rounding of the chin.

Two-piece Genioplasty

For those who are unbothered by the shape of the chin but would like to project the chin to create an elongated shape of the lower face, the author recommends the 2-piece or sliding genioplasty. The 2-piece genioplasty can also be performed for reduction in a setback, but this is not preferred as it causes submental fullness which is unfavorable aesthetically for the patient. In cases that only require reduction, a 1-piece is generally preferred.

While this approach projects the chin and makes it more prominent, it is used in some cases for transfeminine patients seeking to correct microgenia. The projected chin does elongate the lower third of the face. This may create the appearance of a more slender and narrow lower face, despite the fact that the chin is in fact, larger. The senior author informs the patient that osseous advancement genioplasty is preferred to the chin implant, as it allows for specific alterations to the shape and structure of the chin. The advancement osseous genioplasty also provides the added benefit of improving submental fullness (double chin) as it advances soft tissue as well. In addition to the cosmetic benefits, patients may experience some relief from snoring and/or sleep apnea, as advancing the attached glossal muscles alleviates some obstruction from the airway passage from the posterior pharynx.

Three-piece Genioplasty

The 3-piece genioplasty more extensively *narrows* the appearance of the chin and contours it

into the shape of a V. This specific form of genioplasty is able to reduce the width and height of the chin. The 3-piece genioplasty is thus the procedure most often requested by transfeminine patients as it not only narrows the chin but also changes the shape from wide and square to narrow and pointed. For those that request both a dramatic reduction in the projection and shape of the chin, the senior author recommends the 3-piece genioplasty as it is able to narrow and shape the chin and set in a new position as desired.

Jaw Reduction

In addition to the narrowing or rounding of the chin, transfeminine patients often cite the desire to reduce the squareness of their jaw angles. Thus the 3-piece genioplasty is often accompanied by mandibular angle reduction in a set of procedures collectively termed V-line surgery. A thorough discussion of the evaluation, technique, and aesthetics of mandibular angle reduction is beyond the scope of this article and will be covered in detail in a separate article.

It is important to note, that while surgeons differentiate surgery on the chin from surgery on the mandibular angles, patients do not. In the senior author's experience, when patients request "jaw reduction" or state that their jaws are "too big," they most often point to their chin and the adjacent body of the mandible. A recent study showed no significant differences in jaw angle between men and women.[16] Given this information, many patients may achieve a feminine look without altering the mandibular angles. While jaw angle reduction may be necessary to treat dysphoria and/or feminize the face of some with a significantly flared mandibular angle, often a genioplasty alone is sufficient to create a softer, more feminine lower face.

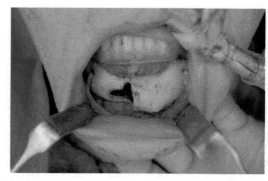

Fig. 5. Side-by-side comparison of the difference in shape and anterior projection of the burred right side compared to the unburred left side.

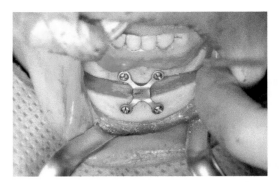

Fig. 6. Anteriorly plated inferior portion of the mandible.

Surgical Technique

The osseous genioplasty is performed under general anesthesia as the procedure necessitates the extensive dissection of the tissues of the lower face through an intraoral incision. The incision is made about 3 to 5 mm lateral to the apex of the gingivobuccal sulcus, on the labial side. Extending the incision slightly laterally ensures that a sufficient cuff of mucosa remains for adequate closure. The incision is approximately from canine to canine, or as wide as needed to visualize the mental foramen and the mental nerve bilaterally. The mentalis muscles are divided as the dissection extends inferiorly. A thick cuff of mentalis muscle remains attached to the mandibular symphysis, allowing for later resuspension. The subperiosteal dissection continues inferiorly to the mental protuberances, and then extends laterally to locate and protect the mental foramen and mental nerve. Additional inferolateral dissection is performed to allow for a longer osteotomy and minimize mandibular notching. To maintain vascular integrity, the soft tissue at the inferior edge of the mandible should remain intact and attached to the periosteum. To avoid asymmetries, the skeletal midline is marked via a reference line drawn down the dental midline.

One-piece Genioplasty

The 1-piece genioplasty consists of surface reduction of the bone. This can be done in a variety of ways. The senior author prefers a 4.0 mm oval solid carbide burr, commonly referred to as an "egg burr." The amount of reduction is limited by the thickness of the cortical bone anteriorly. A moderate amount of cancellous bone may also be burred as long as there is sufficient bone posteriorly and laterally to maintain structural integrity (**Figs. 4 and 5**).

Two-piece Genioplasty

The 2-piece genioplasty or sliding genioplasty, as described in literature, involves a single horizontal osteotomy performed at least 5 mm inferior to the mental foramen in order to protect the integrity of the mental nerve. For transfeminine patients that want to reduce the anterior projection of their chin through this procedure, the bone is replaced posteriorly and secured via titanium step-off plates in a recessed position.

In the advancement 2-piece genioplasty, the cut portion of the mandible is advanced forward and fixed to the superior portion of the mandible via titanium step-off plates (**Fig. 6**). The degree of anterior projection for this procedure is limited by the amount that the bone can be advanced while still offering some overlap between the inferior and superior portions. This overlap allows for osseous regrowth following surgery and minimizes the risk of nonunion.

Three-piece Genioplasty

Without preoperative virtual surgical planning, the osteotomies are planned and marked intraoperatively once the entire bone is exposed. The senior author uses #2 pencils which are sterilized in an autoclave and discarded after use (**Figs. 7 and 8**). First, a horizontal osteotomy at least 5 mm under the mental foramen is marked. This osteotomy may be lower in those with an elongated or

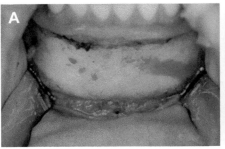
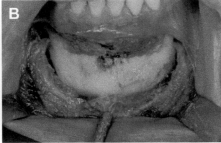

Fig. 7. (*A*), (*B*) Exposed chin with the integrity of the mental nerve preserved bilaterally.

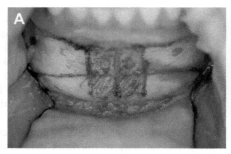
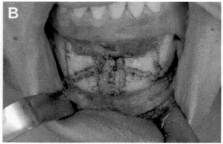

Fig. 8. (*A*), (*B*) Dental midline marking used as a reference for vertical and horizontal osteotomy guideline markings. Medial shaded portion is marked for resection.

large chin, and refining the resulting step-off is a lower risk when there is some distance between it and the mental nerve. The decision to perform vertical or angled osteotomies, and the distance between them, is determined by the patient's anatomy and desired outcome. Vertical osteotomies are performed if the patient desires the same vertical height and only wishes to make the shape more narrow (see **Fig. 7**A). Angled osteotomies are made if the patient desires a more narrow and shortened chin (see **Fig. 7**B). The initial horizontal osteotomy is performed as with the 2-piece genioplasty. The senior author will usually leave a portion of the posterior cortex attached in order to keep the bone stable when performing vertical osteotomies. The inferior, detached portion of the mandible is then split via 2, vertical osteotomies. This trisects the bone into 3 portions: 2 lateral portions and one medial portion (**Fig. 9**).

The medial portion is then removed and the lateral portions are brought together medially and fixed to the mandible symphysis with titanium step-off plates. A typical genioplasty plate can be used to project the chin (**Fig. 10**A). In cases where the chin needs to be slightly recessed, the genioplasty plate may be inverted (**Fig. 10**B). In cases where no advancement or recession is needed, the senior author prefers to use 2 box plates (**Fig. 10**C).

Once the bone of the chin is fixed and resecured to the body of the mandible, there are usually step-offs or gaps created in the transition from the newly positioned portion to the rest of the mandible (**Fig. 11**). These are addressed to avoid any palpable or visible lumps or depressions. Depending on the size and shape of the step-off, this may be addressed with a reciprocating saw, ultrasonic cutting device, or electronic rasp. The mental nerve must be visualized, gently retracted, and protected while the area of bone immediately below it is refined. The use of a burr is not recommended here, as there is a tendency to catch soft tissue in such a narrow space that may place the mental nerve at risk.

Once the step-off is addressed, final refinements to the chin are performed. The genioplasty plates are not load-bearing and generally able to be manipulated. They can be bent in vivo to compensate for any repositioning that occurred with the placement of screws. Small gaps will heal with no intervention. For larger gaps, segments of bone fashioned from the resected step off, or from the discarded medial portion can be reappropriated and inserted (**Figs. 12**; **Fig. 14**A) Any rough transitions can be burred down and any smaller gaps can be packed. To create the packing, the removed medial portion of bone is burred to collect the generated bone dust

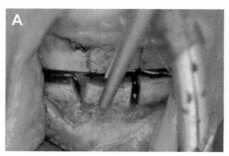
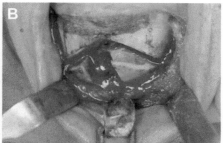

Fig. 9. (*A*), (*B*) Medial section of the detached inferior mandibular portion is removed.

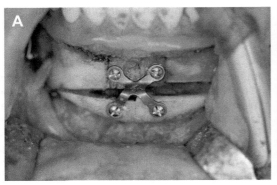
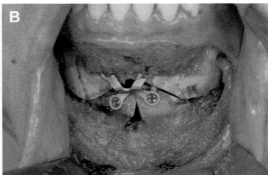
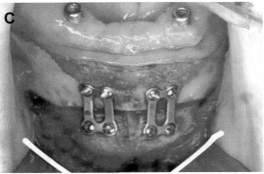

Fig. 10. (A), (B), (C) Lateral sections brought together and secured in an anterior, a posterior, and the same position, respectively, via titanium step-off plates and screws.

(Fig. 13). This bone dust is subsequently mixed with the patient's own blood to create a moldable putty that can be packed into any gaps between the bone and promote osseous regrowth (Fig. 14B).

Resuspension and Closure

If the bone is significantly reduced in the 1-piece genioplasty, there may be a resulting soft tissue excess. In these cases the senior author will often drill bilateral bone tunnels in the inferior cortex to resuspend the chin pad and surrounding soft tissues (Figs. 15–18). This is done in addition to the resuspension of the mentalis muscle. Spreading and securing the soft tissue helps control the shape of the chin and prevents ptosis over time. Despite the bone appearing very flat, when the chin pad is redraped, the resulting chin appears round and recessed from the outside.

In all cases, the mentalis muscle is resuspended via bilateral 3 to 0 vicryl sutures. A large bite is taken along the cut edge of the muscle in the chin pad and sewn to the cuff of the remaining

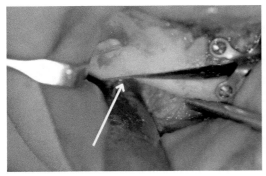

Fig. 11. Step-off deformity created by newly, anteriorly plated inferior mandibular section.

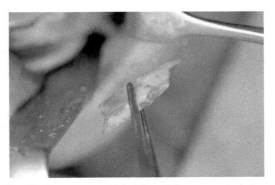

Fig. 12. Bone segment fashioned from resected step-off, superolateral to the horizontal osteotomy.

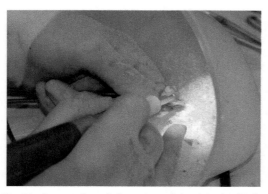

Fig. 13. Resected medial portion of the detached inferior mandibular section burred to collect bone dust.

muscle below the dentition. This resuspension of the mentalis is necessary for all 3 types of genioplasty to anchor the chin pad upwards and minimize the risk of chin ptosis. The mucosal incision is likewise sutured, usually with a 4 to 0 chromic suture. In cases of a big bony reduction, there may be a mismatch between the resuspended labial mucosa and the gingival mucosa. This may require a reduction of the gingivobuccal sulcus length, by trimming the gingival mucosa.

RESULTS
Case Study 1

A 35-year-old who underwent a 1-piece genioplasty to reduce the anterior projection of her chin. Additionally, buccal fat pad removal and helium plasma skin tightening to the neck was performed.

Case Study 2

■

Case Study 3

A 33-year-old who underwent a 3-piece genioplasty with narrowing and advancement. In addition, she

underwent tracheal shave, fat grafting to the malar fat pads, rhinoplasty, and buccal fat pad removal.

Postoperative Management

Immediately postoperatively, patients are dressed in a compression dressing to support the chin and minimize the risk of submental seroma or hematoma formation. Patients are initially wrapped with fluffs, kerlix, and an ace bandage. They are seen on postoperative day 1, and the dressings are removed. Following this initial postoperative visit, they are changed to an elastic garment that gives compression to the chin, jaw, and neck (as needed). Patients are advised to wear the head wrap for as much time as possible for the first week following surgery, usually 22 hours per day. A second postoperative visit is scheduled for 7 to 10 days after surgery to inspect the mucosal incision, monitor swelling, and answer any questions. After this visit, patients are instructed to wear the compression dressing for 12 hours on and 12 hours off. We have found that while wearing the dressing provides adequate compression for the sake of seroma or hematoma prevention, it also impedes lymphatic drainage. Patients will thus have persistent swelling of the cheeks, around the eyes, and anywhere in the face that is not compressed. Having the dressing off for half the day facilitates natural lymphatic drainage while still providing compression to the jaw/chin at night and reducing swelling. Further, most patients have returned to work after 1 week and are reluctant to wear the compression dressing when appearing in public.

Patients are also advised to expect mental nerve paresthesia due to the necessary dissection and retraction of the nerve required to access the underlying mandible. While patients should expect numbness that subsides over the course of months, it is rare for the mental nerve to be permanently damaged. Although the marginal mandibular

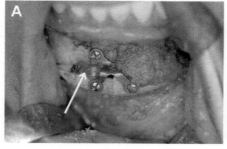
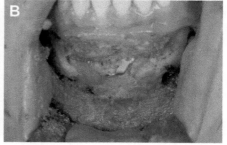

Fig. 14. (A) Bone segment inserted to fill the larger gap with a thick mixture of bone dust and blood having already been applied to the left side, (B) Thick mixture of bone dust and blood used to fill any minor gaps or step-offs between the fixed bone segments.

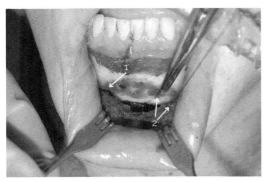

Fig. 15. 1-piece genioplasty with resuspension of the chin pad in progress. 1 - Right side of chin pad suspended through a tunnel burred in the surface of the bone 2 - Left side of chin pad in the process of resuspension through the bone tunnel.

branch of the facial nerve is not in the plane of dissection, neurapraxia is possible. This may be caused by stretch injury during retraction or overzealous cauterization of blood vessels in the soft

tissue. This injury may also take months to return to full function, but permanent injury is rare.

COMPLICATIONS AND MANAGEMENT
Patient Satisfaction

As with any elective cosmetic procedure, there is no guarantee that the surgeon will achieve the desired aesthetic results. Managing patient expectations preoperatively is key to a successful surgery that includes a happy patient. Preoperative counseling includes highlighting existing asymmetries and irregularities, describing the expected outcome, and clearly stating the limitations of the procedure. All humans have some facial asymmetry, some more prominent than others. Pointing out preexisting asymmetries and irregularities is necessary preoperatively, as patients will often scrutinize their facial appearance after surgery. With close scrutiny, they will often notice preexisting features as if they were new and may assume the fault of their surgeon. A gentle and guided

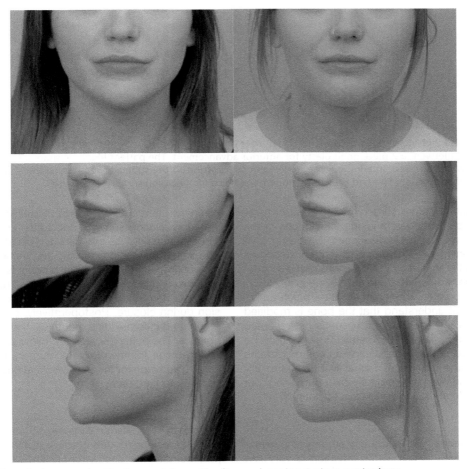

Fig. 16. Case 1 photographed before and 1 month after undergoing 1-piece genioplasty.

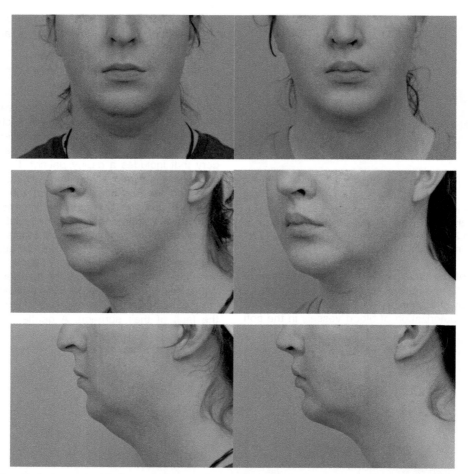

Fig. 17. Case 2 photographed before and 1 year after undergoing 2-piece advancement genioplasty. A 31-year-old who underwent a 2-piece genioplasty for anterior advancement. The patient liked the shape of her chin but felt it was too recessed. In addition, she underwent fat grafting to the submalar area, rhinoplasty, lip lift, and submental liposuction. She had previously undergone voice feminization surgery elsewhere.

conversation before surgery can prevent or minimize these misunderstandings. Limitations of the surgery must also be discussed. Following a 3-piece genioplasty, the degree that the chin comes to a point is limited by the thickness of the soft tissue redraped over it. If the soft tissue is too thick, then the pointed appearance will be blunted. Patients must understand that the bone is modified in genioplasty, but the soft tissue is not resected and will stay largely the same. Patients may be counseled about options such as energy devices to shrink the soft tissue, dermal filler to create definition, and neurotoxin to help skin puckering, but must understand there still exist limitations.

Infection

While infection is a risk of any surgery, the senior author's experience is that infection is very low with genioplasties. In this practice, patients are given the standard peri-operative antibiotics intravenously. During surgery, antibiotics are used in the irrigation fluid, usually clindamycin (depending on availability). Before mixing the antibiotics vial into the irrigation fluid, a small amount is set aside and mixed into a more concentrated solution. This concentrated solution is distributed into the incision during closure. Postoperatively, patients are prescribed chlorhexidine mouthwash and oral antibiotics. The patient is seen for follow-up, virtually or in person for months after surgery to ensure healing and monitor for any complications or infection due to hardware.

Seroma or Hematoma

Despite the vascularity of the region and the blood loss that may occur during surgery of the chin and jaw, hematomas and seromas are rare. Proper postoperative care may minimize risk. Patients

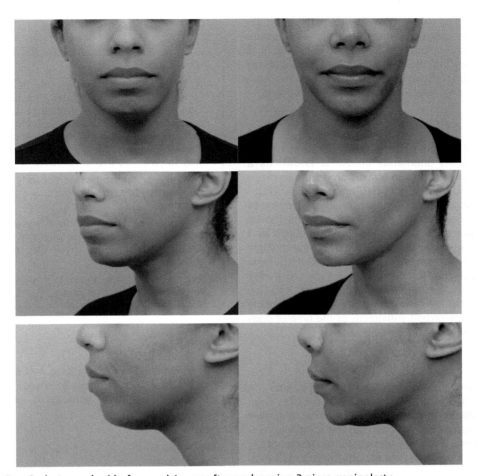

Fig. 18. Case 3 photographed before and 1 year after undergoing 3-piece genioplasty.

are instructed to sleep with their heads elevated and use the provided compression head wrap. If a seroma or hematoma does occur, it can be evacuated by opening a portion of the mucosal incision or through needle aspiration. These patients should be monitored longitudinally with extra postoperative visits as needed. In the case of secondary underlying scar tissue formation, the scar tissue can be treated with a series of 1:1 triamcinolone acetonide 40 Mg/ML injectable suspension and fluorouracil injection to inhibit and break down scar tissue formation.

Submental Fullness

The most notable downside of reduction genioplasty is potential submental fullness and jowling due to the reduced bone volume and mismatch created between the soft tissue and the bone. The degree of this postoperative laxity depends on the quality and elasticity of each patient's tissue, submental fat, and degree of reduction. As mentioned previously, a genioplasty that sets back the bone will create submental fullness and is not commonly performed for greater than 2 mm of reduction. Even without a setback, patients should expect submental fullness for several months as persistent swelling remains in the submental area after surgery.

Any persistent resulting submental fullness and tissue laxity can be addressed with soft tissue interventions such as energy devices, filler, and submental liposuction. In this practice, we offer helium plasma radiofrequency for young patients with good skin elasticity. For older patients who present with skin laxity preoperatively, a facelift is usually recommended. The senior author generally recommends addressing the soft tissue concerns 6 to 12 months postoperatively. This allows for a substantial degree of swelling to be resolved, and areas needing lifting or tightening to be clearly identified. While the energy device can be used at the same time of the surgery, it is generally recommended to wait the standard course of 6 to

12 months as the significant swelling following the procedure may reduce the quality of the soft tissue outcomes. For patients who need a facelift, it is even more important to stage the procedure, as the multiple planes of dissection over the chin and jaw may create complications with healing.

LIP OR CHIN PTOSIS

Ptosis of the chin pad and soft tissue with flattening of the submental crease is known as a "witch's chin" and can result from failure to properly resuspend the chin pad upon closure. Damage to the mentalis muscle or loss of mentalis function can cause lip ptosis, where the red lip folds outward exposing the lower dentition and gums. This repair is very difficult and the multiple steps required are beyond the scope of this article. This ptosis may not present for several years after genioplasty, further complicating repair. The key point is that resuspension of the mentalis muscle must be performed sufficiently at the time of original surgery.

SUMMARY

The osseous genioplasty can be used to alter the appearance of the chin in all 3 dimensions. Chin augmentation through a chin implant can only alter the appearance of the chin with the addition of volume. This is usually in contrast to the desires of the female transgender patient, who wishes to reduce the size or square shape of her chin. The 3 variations of osseous genioplasty described in this article offer solutions that can be tailored to address different aesthetic concerns. The 1-piece genioplasty allows for deprojection and rounding of the chin. 2-piece genioplasty allows for significant projection of the chin without adding lateral volume. The 3-piece genioplasty can be used to alter the chin in 3 planes; it can narrow the chin, and shorten the chin while advancing, reducing, or maintaining the horizontal position. Adequate resuspension of the mentalis muscle is key to preventing chin and lip ptosis postoperatively.

Patients are generally satisfied with the aesthetic results of an osseous genioplasty and note the marked enhancement of femininity that the procedure offers. The change in the chin shape is often enough to soften and feminize the entire lower face, without altering the angle of the mandible. In the senior author's experience, the most common complaint of postgenioplasty patients is lower lip paresthesia due to neuropraxia of the mental nerve. Proper preoperative counseling and managing expectations are key to ensuring patient satisfaction.

CLINICS CARE POINTS

- A traditionally masculine chin is broader, wider, taller, and has greater anterior projection which contributes to a larger and more square appearance. A feminine chin is typically narrower, more pointed, tapered, and shorter. Genioplasty is a safe and effective way to feminize the lower face.
- The type or method of genioplasty depends on the patient's current anatomy and desired outcome.
- Care must be taken to identify and protect the mental nerve bilaterally but patients should still expect lower lip numbness postoperatively.
- Resuspension of the mentalis muscle is crucial to prevent future chin ptosis.

DISCLOSURE

Dr R.E. Rodman is a consultant and speaker for Apyx Medical. All references to energy devices in this article have been generalized to preserve anonymity.

REFERENCES

1. Bruce V, Burton AM, Hanna E, et al. Sex discrimination: How do we tell the difference between male and female faces? Perception 1993;22(2):131–52.
2. Ousterhout DK. Facial feminization surgery: a guide for the transgendered woman. Addicus Books; 2010.
3. Park S, Noh JH. Importance of the chin in lower facial contour: Narrowing genioplasty to achieve a feminine and slim lower face. Plast Reconstr Surg 2008;122(1):261–8.
4. Lee TS, Kim HY, Kim TH, et al. Contouring of the lower face by a novel method of narrowing and lengthening genioplasty. Plast Reconstr Surg 2014; 133(3). https://doi.org/10.1097/01.prs.0000438054.21634.4a.
5. Hsu Y-c, Li J, Hu J, et al. Correction of square jaw with low angles using mandibular "V-line" ostectomy combined with outer cortex ostectomy. Oral Surgery, Oral Medicine, Oral Pathology, Oral Radiology, and Endodontology 2010;109(2):197–202.
6. Hofer O. Operation der prognathie und mikrogenie. Deutsche Zahn Mund und Kieferheilkunde 1942;9:121.
7. Trauner R, Obwegeser H. The surgical correction of mandibular prognathism and Retrognathia with

consideration of genioplasty. Oral Surg Oral Med Oral Pathol 1957;10(7):677–89.

8. Spiessl B. Internal fixation of the mandible. Berlin: Springer Verlag; 2012. https://doi.org/10.1007/978-3-642-71034-6.

9. Xia J, Ip HHS, Samman N, et al. Computer-assisted three-dimensional surgical planning and simulation: 3D virtual Osteotomy. Int J Oral Maxillofac Surg 2000;29(1):11–7.

10. Olszewski R, Reychler H. Computer-assisted genioplasty: Three-dimensional planning and transfer to the Operating Theatre. Int J Oral Maxillofac Surg 2009;38(5):474.

11. Efanov JI, Roy A-A, Huang KN, et al. Virtual Surgical Planning. Plastic and Reconstructive Surgery - Global Open 2018;6(1). https://doi.org/10.1097/gox.0000000000001443.

12. Lesavoy MA, Creasman C, Schwartz RJ. A technique for correcting witch's chin deformity. Plast Reconstr Surg 1996;97(4):842–6.

13. Hwang K, Lee WJ, Song YB, et al. Vulnerability of the inferior alveolar nerve and mental nerve during GENIOPLASTY: An anatomic study. J Craniofac Surg 2005;16(1):10–4.

14. Chang EW, Lam SM, Karen M, et al. Sliding genioplasty for correction of Chin abnormalities. Arch Facial Plast Surg 2001;3(1):8–15.

15. Hoang H, Bertrand AA, Hu AC, et al. Simplifying facial feminization surgery using virtual modeling on the Female Skull. Plastic and Reconstructive Surgery - Global Open 2020;8(3). https://doi.org/10.1097/gox.0000000000002618.

16. Bannister JJ, Juszczak H, Aponte JD, et al. Sex differences in adult facial three-dimensional morphology: Application to gender-affirming facial surgery. Facial Plastic Surgery & Aesthetic Medicine 2022;24(S2). https://doi.org/10.1089/fpsam.2021.0301.

Moving?

Make sure your subscription moves with you!

To notify us of your new address, find your **Clinics Account Number** (located on your mailing label above your name), and contact customer service at:

Email: journalscustomerservice-usa@elsevier.com

800-654-2452 (subscribers in the U.S. & Canada)
314-447-8871 (subscribers outside of the U.S. & Canada)

Fax number: 314-447-8029

Elsevier Health Sciences Division
Subscription Customer Service
3251 Riverport Lane
Maryland Heights, MO 63043

*To ensure uninterrupted delivery of your subscription, please notify us at least 4 weeks in advance of move.

9780443182600